THE MRCGP
EXAMINATION

THE MRCGP EXAMINATION

A comprehensive guide to preparation and passing

Squadron-Leader A. J. MOULDS, M.R.C.G.P., R.A.F.
Assistant Tutor in General Practice, RAM College, Millbank

Lieutenant-Colonel T. A. Bouchier Hayes, M.R.C.G.P., R.A.M.C.
Tutor in General Practice, RAM College, Millbank

Colonel K. H. M. Young, O.B.E., F.R.C.G.P., R.A.M.C.
Adviser in General Practice to the Director General Army Medical Services

MTPPRESS LIMITED *International Medical Publishers*

Published by
MTP Press Limited
Falcon House
Cable Street
Lancaster, England

Copyright © 1978 MTP Press Limited

Reprinted 1985

ISBN: 0 85200 238–6

Printed in Great Britain by
Redwood Burn Limited, Trowbridge, Wiltshire

Contents

Foreword: John FRY   vii

1   The MRCGP examination: *A. J. Moulds*   1

2   The modified essay question paper or MEQ: *A. J. Moulds*   7

3   The traditional essay question paper or TEQ: *T. A. Bouchier Hayes*   11

4   The multiple-choice question paper or MCQ: *A. J. Moulds*   15

5   The oral examination and log diary: *K. Young*   21

6   The problem-solving oral: *K. Young*   37

7   Vital statistics: *A. J. Moulds*   45

8   Sources of information: *T. A. Bouchier Hayes*   49

9   Work plan: *A. J. Moulds*   55

10   Mock examination and answers: MEQ; TEQ; MCQ: *T. A. Bouchier Hayes and A. J. Moulds*   57

Foreword

JOHN FRY

All examinations create problems and stresses in examinees. The examination for the Membership of the Royal College of General Practitioners is no exception. Although the examiners state that their objectives are to pass candidates wherever and whenever possible, nevertheless the failure rate remains consistently at 30% plus of those taking the examination.

The reasons for failure fall into a number of groups. The candidate may, through over-confidence, not have prepared for the examination. He may have assumed that it is not necessary to read, learn and digest data, facts and experience on general practice. How wrong that is, he will discover when he sits the exam. There is much reading and learning to be done for the MRCGP. The candidate must do this himself with the help of a tutor.

Another reason is unfamiliarity with the special nature and format of the MRCGP examination – with MCQs, MEQ, TEQ and oral tests.

This book has been written to help candidates with the latter problems. It has been designed to help prepare and familiarise the candidates with the various parts of the exam. It cannot, and is not intended to, serve as a textbook, or as a mine of information, for possible questions. The candidate must read the current books on general practice or general medicine, on community care and on other subjects. He must read the current journals and in particular the College publications. The book will, however, show the candidate how the questions are presented, how the examiners expect the answers to be given and how the marking is carried out.

The authors have been the organisers of some of the most successful courses for the MRCGP exam. They have achieved very high pass-rates in those prospective candidates who attended their courses. They are all serving officers in Her Majesty's Forces; a most unusual qualification for authors of a book.

It is because the Forces were faced with the problems of providing care for families and with creating the speciality of general practice that they have become so experienced and expert. The Forces had to train and educate family doctors. They believed that Membership of the Royal College of General Practitioners was an essential criterion for good general practitioners. They set out to encourage officers to prepare and sit for the MRCGP, and they assist them with courses held at Millbank twice a year.

The book demonstrates their effective methods; it is dedicated to future candidates for MRCGP and to the future advancement of the College.

I am sure that if future candidates for MRCGP read, learn and digest the lessons within this book, the challenges of the examination will become less hazardous and the actual tests may become actually enjoyable!

1
The MRCGP Examination

A. J. MOULDS

The Royal College of General Practitioners was established in 1952. The introduction of the examination was in 1966, and in 1969 it became the only portal of entry to College membership. In 1969, 82 candidates sat the exam (78% passing) while in 1977, 828 candidates sat (66% passing). Obviously the exam is providing a much-needed postgraduate goal for General Practitioners, and the majority sitting are still established principals rather than vocational trainees. The exam is designed to test the minimum standards of competence required to be shown by a principal in general practice. It covers the main content of general practice and is not too difficult if properly prepared for. There is no policy to keep College membership down, and if all candidates were equally good then all would pass! Unfortunately all candidates are not equally good and about 20% will not get past the written stage of the exam; while up to another 20% will fail at the orals.

The aims of this book are:

A. to familiarise the candidate with the format and style of the exam;
B. to give an understanding of the methods of assessment used;
C. to help the candidate present his knowledge without fear of underachieving because of poor or faulty exam technique;
D. to give a guide to preparation.

This book will not help someone without the prerequisite clinical knowledge and competence to pass, but it will help those with such knowledge not to fail. It is not a substitute for study and individual effort but an adjunct to it.

1

ELIGIBILITY TO SIT THE EXAM
A candidate must be either:

1. a vocational trainee who has finished (or is within 8 weeks of finishing) a recognised 3-year course of vocational training for general practice; *or*
2. a fully registered Medical Practitioner for a minimum of 4 years (at least 2 of which must have been in general practice).

If you have any doubts about your eligibility then contact the College who obviously are the definitive authority.

APPLICATION FORMS
These are obtainable from: The Membership Secretary, The Royal College of General Practitioners, 14 Princess Gate, Hyde Park, London SW7 1PU. (Telephone: 01 584 6262).

Remember that, although the exam may be in May or November, the closing date for applications is 6 weeks before the written papers. Plan well ahead, especially as increasing applications may make it necessary for the College to limit the total number of candidates at any one sitting. With the application form the College sends an extremely helpful booklet of explanatory notes, a reprint of an article by Dr J. Howie on the exam (although parts of this article are out of date it gives some useful advice and is well worth reading), and the current schedule of exam and membership fees.

DATES AND VENUES
The written parts of the exam are held in May and late October/early November in London, Leeds, Manchester, Edinburgh, Newcastle, Aberdeen, Cardiff, Belfast and Dublin – subject to demand. The orals are in late June/early July and December (about 6 weeks after the writtens) in either London or Edinburgh.

FORMAT
Part I of the exam consists of three written papers which are all completed in one day. Generally the modified essay and traditional essay papers are done in the morning, with the multiple-choice questionnaire in the afternoon.

The times allotted are:

A. Modified essay question paper (MEQ) 45 minutes or 1 hour.
B. Traditional essay paper (TEQ) 90 minutes
C. Multiple-choice questionnaire(MCQ) 3 hours.

Part II of the exam consists of two consecutive orals, each lasting approximately 30 minutes. (A recent College decision has in fact shortened the orals to 25 minutes each with 5 minutes for the examiners to discuss the candidates' performance.)

D. Practice Log Diary oral.
E. Problem-solving oral.

All these parts of the exam are fully explored in their individual chapters. They complement each other in testing the knowledge,

Table 1

	Knowledge	Interview skills	Problem-solving skills	Technical skills	Attitudes
MCQ	+++				
MEQ	+		+++		+
TEQ	++		++		+
Log Diary oral	+	++	++		++
Problem-solving oral	+	++	++		++

skills and attitudes of the candidate in 'whole person' medicine, and Table 1 gives a rough idea of their varying emphasis. Without clinicals, technical skills cannot really be tested, although possibly at some time in the future the College will introduce patients into the exam.

MARKING
All five parts of the exam have equal weighting, and to pass overall a candidate must score an average of about 55%. Any candidate who is invited to come for the orals has a chance of passing, although he will be given no other indication of what his mark may be; also, the oral examiners are not aware of the written marks while oralling and only know that the candidate could pass overall.

The examiners are all active General Practitioners drawn from all faculties of the College and so come from every area of Great Britain. They sit the written papers themselves to help produce the consensus answers which are used as the standard for marking. This breadth of opinion allows the marking schedules to reflect current practice throughout the country and means that no individual examiner can introduce unusual or controversial views into the marking.

Each part of the exam is separately marked by two examiners (apart from the MCQ which is marked by computer scanning) whose assessments of the candidate's performance have to be in fairly close agreement. If they are not then the paper is remarked and possibly referred to a third examiner.

All in all this is a genuinely fair system, with any doubts or disagreements between examiners being referred to more senior examiners and no candidate failing without serious thought having been given to his performance.

AREAS OF KNOWLEDGE TESTED

'The Future General Practitioner – Learning and Teaching' constructed a concise definition of the General Practitioner's job and also elucidated the content of general practice. It is on these foundations that the examination is based.

Job definition:

The General Practitioner is a doctor who provides personal, primary and continuing medical care to individuals and families. He may attend his patients in their homes, in his consulting room or sometimes in hospital. He accepts the responsibility for making an initial decision on every problem his patient may present to him, consulting with Specialists when he thinks it appropriate to do so. He will usually work in a group with other General Practitioners, from premises that are built or modified for the purpose, with the help of paramedical colleagues, adequate secretarial staff and all the equipment that is necessary. His diagnosis will be composed in physical, psychological and social terms. He will intervene educationally, preventatively and therapeutically to promote his patient's health.

The educational content of general practice needing to be studied for the examination covers broadly:

1. diagnosis, management and prevention of disease in general practice;
2. health and health education;
3. normal and abnormal human development from conception

to death and how it affects diagnosis and management of disease;

4. psychological/behavioural factors as they affect the presentation and management of disease;
5. the relevance of sociology and epidemiology to medical care;
6. the organization of medical and paramedical services in Great Britain and abroad;
7. practice organisation and administration;
8. recent developments in the evolution of general practice.

This is a substantial area of knowledge but only reflects the essential knowledge needed for good general practice.

Apart from general learning each candidate will have weaknesses that need to be strengthened before the exam. Service candidates, for example, will need to cover geriatrics and practice organisation. New town doctors may also need to cover geriatrics, while those with large geriatric populations may need to brush up their paediatrics, and so on!

RESULTS

All candidates are notified, by letter, of their results. About 3–4 weeks after the writtens (it seems much longer!), the candidate will either be informed that he has already failed and does not need to come for orals, or that he has performed sufficiently well to reach the orals. He will then be given his oral date and time. (After the candidate's application form has been processed a provisional oral date is allocated. At this time the candidate is also sent details of the written timetable and a log diary to fill in.)

After the orals the final results are sent out as quickly as possible and nearly everyone will know their result within a week at most. Those who pass are invited to become members of the College, on payment of an additional fee. Those who fail are allowed to re-sit at a lower rate in the future. Anyone who does fail should write to the College for further information about their areas of weakness, as the College is quite prepared to give an assessment of the candidate's performance.

A few will pass with distinction, which means that the average of their marks, in all five parts of the examination, is greater than 70%. The best of these, over the year, is awarded a prize by the College.

2

The Modified Essay Question Paper or MEQ

A. J. MOULDS

The MEQ broadly examines diagnostic ability and clinical management. It is very much the College's 'baby', having been developed from the patient-management type of question used in some overseas examinations. As it lends itself particularly to testing in a general practice situation the examination style is not commonly used in other United Kingdom examinations, and many candidates are likely to be unfamiliar with it.

Basically the MEQ is constructed from the case-records of a patient or, more usually, a family in one of the examiner's practices. Background information is given and then the clinical picture, of an illness or illnesses, is unfolded. Additional information is given as the story progresses, but at each stage of the development the candidate is required to answer a series of questions. This represents the general practitioner's method of working with decisions being made, at a given point in time, on the basis of the information available. The ongoing commitment is also recognised, with continual monitoring bringing to light further information, which may lead to a review of the actions taken.

A typical MEQ might develop in the following manner:

Mrs Pink, a 47-year-old housewife, has recently moved into your practice area. Her 50-year-old husband is a GPO telephone engineer and she has three children aged 4, 14 and 17. The youngest, David, suffers from Downs' syndrome.

Mrs Pink complains that she is finding it increasingly difficult to cope with David.

1. What agencies could you enlist to help with David?

A few weeks later Mrs Pink returns to you complaining of headaches.

7

2. (a) What information do you want from her to help you reach a diagnosis?

(b) What are the four most likely causes of headaches?

(c) What is the most likely cause in this case?

(d) Discuss your initial management.

Her headaches decrease but she complains of increasing depression.

3. What two factors would help you most in assessing the severity of her depression?

You decide that she is clinically depressed and needs treatment.

4. Discuss under four headings the next steps in your management.

You decide to prescribe a tricyclic antidepressant.

5. (a) Describe your dosage plan.

(b) Discuss the possible side-effects of tricyclic antidepressants.

The paper could then be developed in a variety of ways; e.g.:

Mr Pink may have a myocardial infarction or develop an ulcer.
David may develop asthma.
Mrs Pink may become menopausal or find a lump in her breast.
One of the teenagers may have a grand mal fit; etc.

The paper comes in the form of a loose-leaf book with the questions fairly evenly spaced out on their own pages. After each question blank spaces are left for the candidate to write in his answer.

Different questions may be marked by different examiners, and all questions do not necessarily carry the same number of marks. Common sense would tell you, for example, that Q3 would have less marks than Q2.

The number of questions and time allowed for them does vary although it is most likely to be either twelve questions in 60 minutes or nine in 45 minutes. The actual timing involved is made very clear in the instructions, given immediately prior to the paper, and an indication is also given, on the paper, of how far on you are.

These points will be more readily understood once you have done the mock MEQ.

There are many points to note when doing the MEQ:

A. Read the instructions carefully before you start. Be sure you know exactly what is being asked of you.

B. Do not look through the whole MEQ before starting. Take each question as it comes. Your practical approach to a developing general practice situation is being tested, and you must try to imagine yourself in your own surgery actually dealing with the problem. If you look ahead your weighting of the probabilities may well be altered; e.g.:

> A man presents with a headache and is eventually found to have a cerebral neoplasm. If you have read ahead and seen the 'answer' then you will be influenced by it. You may put down skull x-ray or EEG as one of your first investigations when, patently, in general practice cerebral neoplasm as a cause of headache is very rare and would tend not to figure highly in your initial differential diagnosis.

If you put down treatment or investigations that are inappropriate for the information you have, then that is as bad as missing them out when they are appropriate!

C. Do not go back and alter your answers once you have completed the whole MEQ. The reasons for this are the same as given for not reading ahead; your perspective has been altered by your knowledge of the outcome.

D. Notwithstanding point **C**, there may be a question where you have gone off the track and subsequent information gives you a chance to correct yourself. If, for example, in Q4 drug therapy was not one of your headings, with tricyclic antidepressants getting the main mention, then Q5 would justify your re-thinking of your answer.

E. Read the information and the questions carefully. This is stating the obvious but some candidates do tend to answer the question they would like to have been asked rather than the actual question!

F. Answer clearly, briefly and concisely.

G. Obey instructions that are given in the question. If the question says 'List four causes' then list four and four only, as no credit will be given for any elaboration or extra points you make.

H. Time is crucial and the paper must be approached at a canter rather than a stroll! Many candidates will not finish in time unless they get in some practice before the examination. Past *Updates* are a good source, as is the College, which will send out past MEQs on request.

The marking of the MEQ is based on the examiners' consensus answers with some answers being 'more correct' than others and attracting extra marks. Taking Q3 as an example you are asked for the two factors that would help you most in assessing the severity of depression. Now clearly there are more than two possibilities here and the marking schedule might be:

Suicide risk	3
Sleep disturbance	2
Diurnal variation of mood	2
Non-verbal clues at interview	2
Loss of libido	1
Physical symptoms	1
Past history of depression	1

With a total of 5 for the question anyone putting down suicide risk has already scored 3, and even if your weighting is not the same as the examiner's you can still score 4 out of 5.

Note again that as you are asked for two possibilities then only two will be marked, and if you put down all the possibilities you would only get the marks appropriate to your first two. As with the other papers in the examination the marking system is very fair and has the big advantage of giving credit to differing answers rather than having one right answer with all the others wrong.

Making up an MEQ is fairly difficult, but getting the consensus answers, in the same way as the College does, is very difficult indeed. Therefore we are very grateful to the College for allowing us to use one of their old MEQs and its consensus marking schedule. Reading it is not nearly as valuable as doing it, and so we are using it as the Mock MEQ.

Do it under exam conditions and mark it carefully. The marking schedule will teach you as much about how to approach the MEQ as this chapter has!

3

Traditional Essay Question Paper or TEQ

T. A. BOUCHIER HAYES

The traditional essay question paper is the most underrated part of the MRCGP examination, although it carries marks equal to the other papers. All postgraduate doctors, from their medical student days, are familiar with the TEQ and perhaps this familiarity means that not enough attention is devoted to this one part of the examination where 'spotting' is possible. The TEQ contains three essay questions all of which have to be answered in the course of $1\frac{1}{2}$ hours. The object of the TEQ is to allow the candidate the opportunity to show his knowledge of the subject and how he can construct an answer that is well set out, logical, practical and to the point. Topics may be administrative (health centres, Court report), clinical (carcinoma of the cervix, hypertension) or a mixture of physical and psychosocial (enuresis, alcoholism). Usually, but by no means invariably, there is one question from each of these broad groupings in the paper. Often the questions are related to current debate or 'talking points' or to an important report or committee, and candidates who are not *au fait* with the topical issues have only themselves to blame if they find a question they can answer only in the vaguest terms.

PLANNING THE WHOLE PAPER
You are asked to answer three questions in $1\frac{1}{2}$ hours. There is no choice and all questions must be answered. Each question carries equal marks. Read the question carefully; the examiners have reasons for setting the question as it is set out. Do not try to read into it meanings which it does not have. Do not answer 'your own question', thereby bringing in irrelevant matter. A question may bear superficial resemblance to another question which you have revised for the examination, but you will be

11

unwise to give a version of your previously prepared answer. Often all that is required is a re-ordering of your ideas, with the addition of some new material which you already know.

Take a little while to marshall your thoughts and ideas and lay out your answer. Do not start and write without stopping. Answer all the questions and give yourself an equal amount of time for each one. Allow 5 minutes for planning the essay and up to 5 minutes for a revision of the text. This leaves 20 minutes for each question. At a maximum you should be able to write some four hundred words in 20 minutes. Although it is never possible to know an equal amount about each question it is a mistake to 'write off' one of the three questions. However excellent the two fully answered questions, it is rarely possible to reach an overall pass mark if the third question is of a very poor quality.

Clear handwriting is a duty, not simply a virtue. The examiner does not give marks for an illegible script on the basis that, had he been able to read it, the candidate might well have been producing good work. Usually the reverse is true. Bad writing is marked down, because the examiner cannot get at the ideas of the candidate. If you know that your handwriting is difficult to read, choose a fountain pen rather than a ball-point which tends to exaggerate the faults of bad handwriting.

WRITING
Overall structure

The successful essay has a demonstrable shape. There should be a short introduction, sometimes no more than one or two sentences, in which the major themes or arguments to be discussed are outlined. It is a weakness to open simply by re-phrasing the question. Something must be added.

The major part of the essay may be divided up in a number of ways. Each major division should, where possible, be given a clear heading in capitals so that the examiner is made aware of the shape of your plan. For example, if the question asks for the causes and effects of three sorts of events you may decide to make CAUSES and EFFECTS your two headings. Alternatively, you may make headings of the three sorts of EVENTS, listing causes and effects under each.

Finally, there should be a concluding paragraph which does

not just summarise what has gone before, but which makes a further statement or statements about the material covered.

Paragraphs

You should learn to think in paragraphs. Each paragraph should contain the description of one main idea or event, or the working out of one main argument. Often each of the headings or each of the sub-headings will demand a separate paragraph. It is irritating to run a number of ideas together in a long paragraph. Worse still is the habit of producing a paragraph which contains two or three ideas, lengthened by adding sentence after sentence which modifies or amplifies these ideas in random sequence.

Language

Short sentences are easier to understand than long ones, though they may be more difficult to construct. Long and complicated sentences, if they are to be successful, require a fine command of the rules of grammar and a flair for style. Never pad; it gains no extra marks and makes it difficult for the examiner who marks according to a crib. The easier for the examiner to find your ideas, the higher the marks.

Where possible, make clear the sources of your evidence. Quote authors even if you cannot quote papers, books or dates.

The following example of a TEQ marking crib emphasises the above points.

TEQ CRIB
Question 1

A 42-year-old man consults you about a hydrocele. As he is leaving he asks you to check his blood pressure and you find it is 180/110. What would you do? What information will enable you to make a decision about further treatment?

Key factors

Do nothing regarding further investigation or treatment until more readings have been obtained	2 marks
Discover the reason for the question and discuss possible anxieties	1 mark

Collect information on:

Smoking	0.5 marks
Weight	0.5 marks

Family history	0.5 marks
Occupation	0.5 marks
Stress	0.5 marks
Exercise	0.5 marks

If subsequent readings at rest remain at this level:

Examine CVS (including fundi, peripheral pulses)	1 mark
Take blood for FBC, urea, cholesterol	0.5 marks
Do chest x-ray	0.5 marks
Do ECG	0.5 marks
Do MSU	0.5 marks

A further mark is available for general competence, including mention of lipids, IVP, etc. and full explanation to patient.

Conclusion

A satisfactory essay depends on clear presentation, a firm grasp of the material which is presented and a well-produced logical argument. In addition to these basic qualities, an essay of distinction should show a critical evaluation of the material, and some imagination and creativity in the way in which the candidate presents the material, advances an argument or suggests a conclusion.

4

The Multiple-choice Question Paper
or MCQ

A. J. MOULDS

The MCQ is the part of the exam which most of all seeks to test purely factual knowledge. It consists of ninety questions each of which has a stem statement followed by five completions or items requiring true/false/don't know answers. The stem and one item together make up the statement which you have to consider and, when answering, you should disregard all the other items in that question as they have nothing to do with the one you are concentrating on. A total of 450 answers have to be filled in in the 3 hours allotted. This may seem a daunting prospect but in fact the time allowed is more than adequate and many candidates will finish early.

The proportions of the ninety questions devoted to the different areas of general practice knowledge is obviously important. The College give a breakdown of the questions which currently is as shown below.

General Medicine (M)	20
Psychiatry (Ps)	18
Obstetrics and Gynaecology (O)	12
Therapeutics (T)	10
Paediatrics (Pa)	10
Surgical Diagnosis (Su)	5
Ears, Nose & Throat (ENT)	
Ophthalmology (Op)	10
Dermatology (D)	
Community Medicine (CM)	5

This weighting should be borne in mind when deciding your revision timetable and should be reflected in the times you allot for each subject. The question paper itself is in book form and the answers have to be recorded on special sheets which allow com-

15

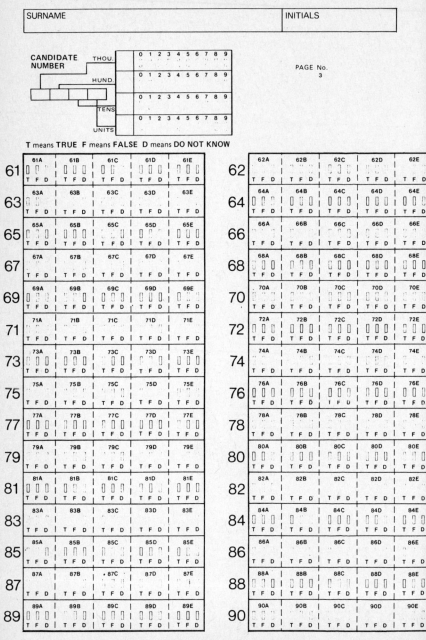

Figure 1   Computer card answer sheet

puter marking (see Figure 1). Each question part has its own true/false/don't know boxes, only one of which has to be shaded in. Remember there is no reason why all the items in a question should not be true or why they should not all be false. A pencil and rubber are provided in the exam, although it is wise to bring your own as well.

By photoelectric scanning the computer will select the most heavily shaded box as the given answer. If you have filled in the wrong box by mistake then you must erase your wrong answer so that its shading is lighter than your final choice. For the same reason the computer will reject any question which has no answer box filled in.

The paper is marked by a negative marking system. Therefore:

a correct answer scores $+1$
an incorrect answer scores -1
a don't know scores 0

This is very important, as guessing is heavily penalised and your approach to your answering should take full account of it. To elaborate, using one question as an example:

MEASLES VACCINATION
A. Should be given in the first year of life.
B. Should not be given to a debilitated child as it would be more likely to develop complications.
C. Is contraindicated in the presence of active eczema.
D. Gives an incidence of serious permanent neurological damage in about 1 per 10^6.
E. Should be modified by simultaneous passive immunization with hyperimmune gamma globulin in children with chronic asthma.

ANSWERS
A. False   Second year of life and if delayed until age 3 then decreased risk of occasional severe reaction.
B. False   Is especially valuable in the debilitated child.
C. False   Smallpox vaccination is contraindicated in the presence of eczema, not measles.
D. True   Much less than the risks of the disease.
E. True   Also in those with bronchiectasis.

So F F F T T   would score   5/5
   F ⚡ F T T   would score   3/5

F X̶ F T X̶   would score   1/5
X̶ X̶ F T X̶   would score   −1/5
D D F T T   would score   3/5

Complete guessing over a negatively marked exam would give 0% (assuming you guessed half right and half wrong) rather than the possible 50% of a non-punitive marking system.

Read every question carefully. This may seem obvious but avoidable errors can occur when a question is read quickly and answered without reflection. On the other hand there will be some questions that you could read forever and still be no nearer an answer, so, mark a 'don't know' and move on to more productive areas.

The time to plan your answering strategy is before the exam rather than during it. Table 2 gives you an idea of what to aim

Table 2

No. True/False answers (out of 450)	Percentage score if ALL are correct	Percentage score if 10 are wrong
225	50	45.5
250	55.5	51
275	61	56.6
300	66.6	62

for. The reason for giving the percentage score if 10 of your answers are wrong is that no-one can be absolutely certain that his answers are correct.

Take the following example:

THE FOLLOWING ARE RECOGNIZED SIDE-EFFECTS OF THE DRUGS NAMED
A. Constipation with magnesium trisilicate.
B. Iron deficiency anaemia with phenytoin.
C. Bradycardia with atropine.
D. Urticaria with aspirin.
E. Megaloblastic anaemia with phenobarbitone.

ANSWERS
A. False   The opposite in fact.
B. False   Megaloblastic anaemia from folic acid deficiency is well recognised.
C. False   Bradycardia is the main indication for its use.
D. True   And asthma in some sensitive people.
E. True   Not as commonly as with phenytoin but it does occur.

Now most people would mark **E** as False and be quite sure that they had gained a mark. By using the second column to gauge your score you allow yourself some leeway for errors.

Some will prefer to go through the paper answering each question in turn, while others will prefer to go quickly through answering all the questions they are sure of and then coming back to think more about the rest. Whichever method you choose is up to you, but it is feasible to go through the paper marking in all the True/False answers you are sure of and then adding them up to see where you stand. If you have below 250 then you would have to guess some, whereas if you have 275 or more you could fill the rest in as 'don't knows' and stop; in between you judge for yourself.

Whatever plan you adopt for yourself, if you finish early it is always worth going over the paper to check you have put down the answers you meant to, and also to ensure you have put the answers in the correct boxes.

At the end of this book there is a mock exam with a ninety-question MCQ. Do it under exam conditions with strict time-keeping and try out your own plan. The content of each question is identified by the letter shown at the start of this chapter, so you can break down your results for each subject and identify your areas of weakness. Hopefully this will be in time for you to take remedial action!

5
The Oral Examination and Log Diary

K. YOUNG

This section of the examination takes place some 6 weeks after the candidate has attempted the written part. The orals are in only two centres – namely Edinburgh and London – and may take a week or more depending on the number of candidates called forward after the papers have been marked. If you are advised to attend for oral examination you should derive some confidence from the fact that you have attained at least a minimally acceptable standard in the writtens and require only to satisfy the examiners to the same degree in your orals.

It must be pointed out, however, that a high level of marks in the papers would not necessarily compensate for failure in one or both orals – i.e. passing the examination is not *just* the attainment of an agreed average mark from the five parts. You must demonstrate a modest competence in all parts, and although failure in one oral may be balanced by a good performance in the other one, too wide a difference in mark between two orals suggests that the examiner's technique and assessment criteria may be at fault!

There are two quite separate oral examinations and each one attracts 20% of the total marks but, for the reason already given, assessment of the candidate's achievements is not based solely on a relatively crude mark count. Each oral take half an hour and each is conducted by two examiners. Thus you meet four examiners in all. The end of the half-hour is signalled by the clash of a gong; a welcome sound indeed!

Oral 1 is based on the Log Diary and the list of patients prepared by the candidate himself, and *Oral 2* is based on problems presented by the examiners. These will be discussed in more details later.

The oral part of the examination is important for the reason

21

that it brings candidate and examiners into direct contact, thus affording the former a chance to express his personality, expertise and compassion and the latter the opportunity to assess these attributes (within the limits of their own skills in the matter). There is no doubt that most candidates find this a very stressful situation and some, as a result, do themselves less than justice. Others, more fortunate perhaps, are stimulated by the challenge and so do better than they might have expected.

The examiners do not try to fail candidates. Indeed it would be fair to state that the majority of them wish to pass the candidate. They are General Practitioners themselves and are mindful of the fact that they are very privileged to be College examiners and that they are assessing their peers and their colleagues who have voluntarily placed themselves in the position of examinee. It cannot be denied that some examiners may be fairly described as hard; a few indeed have been more explicitly if coarsely designated! However, the candidate is well protected from unjust assessment by a system which carefully pairs the examiners and changes them around frequently. There is also the additional safeguard of roving senior examiners or 'wise old men' who keep a close watch on the examiners themselves. So if you are presented with four strangers facing you across the table don't think that you are either a probable failure or a likely distinction candidate – one of the four is probably a trainee examiner and the other is an assessor of the examiners themselves. If then you should still be unfortunate enough to score a mark just below the pass line all is not yet lost! Your examiners must then face a group of two or three senior examiners and justify in detail their reasons for so assessing you. Similarly should you score a very high mark in one oral and a mere pass in the other, both groups of your examiners will be required to defend their assessment of your performance.

Indeed performance in many respects it is, for there is no doubt that appraisal of your demeanour, your personality and powers of expression under the stress of examination, by possibly hostile strangers, plays a large part in the examiner's conscious or unconscious assessment of you. It is, of course, presumed that any General Practitioner, professional that he is, will have achieved a sufficient veneer and sound of confidence to enable him to deal with the infinite variety of patients he will meet in his daily work. There are some who might uncharitably say that if he has not learnt to conceal his doubts and dissimulate his vast areas of ignorance he should not attempt general practice! And however laudable it may be for a General Practitioner to display a proper sense of humility at all times, it must be pointed out that many experienced examiners hold strongly to the idea that a doctor who has not yet learnt that a patient wants his doctor to appear to be confident, wholly absorbed by his disease and yet deeply compassionate and objective, all at the same time, is not yet suitable for membership of the Royal College of General Practitioners. In short you should display to your examiners that although you are a reasonably confident and safe doctor you are at the same time deeply aware of your own limitations in coping with all the trials and tribulations to which humankind is prone.

You are therefore advised to guard against appearing overconfident and above all you must avoid expressing an opinion you cannot substantiate when pressed by an examiner, especially when you suspect that your answer is at variance with the view held by him! Remember that your examiners are experienced General Practitioners and are very skilled in what might be fairly described as either the process of demolishing facades or the exposing of the reality of the candidate's expertise and knowledge rather than his lip service to these basic attributes.

Do not 'dig your own grave' by making statements that you cannot substantiate. For example if you say that you always give iron to menopausal women you must know about the commoner types of anaemia, tests carried out to confirm their presence and the various accepted treatments with their contraindications. Or you may confidently state that you do ECGs on all men above middle age, who present to you with any sort of chest pain or discomfort; but if you do, be prepared to support your opinion and be ready to 'read' an ECG which the examiner may hand you.

On the other hand you may quickly perceive where the examiner is leading you, and if it is not to your taste you should attempt a diversionary ploy which enables you to lead the examiner up paths with which you are more familiar.

Even if the examiner is aware that he is being manipulated it is likely that he will go along with you, so long as the diversion is relevant to the case under discussion.

Before going on to discuss the two orals in more detail let us summarise the points touched on so far.

1. If you are called forward to the oral examination you have succeeded in satisfying the examiners in the written part of the examination and this should give you some measure of confidence.

2. Presuming then that you are in active practice you should possess enough factual knowledge and expertise to satisfy your four examiners – unless you are very unfortunate. Be honest with your examiners but don't admit too hastily to total ignorance until you are quite clear about the question. This you can only do by asking that the question be repeated or rephrased but do not overdo this lest you irritate the examiner and make him think that you are merely stalling.

3. A leaven of humour goes a long way but it should never become facetious, and it is prudent to laugh at the examiner's jokes even if the humour escapes you!

4. Do not be afraid to hold to an opinion at variance with that (apparently) irrefutably held by your examiner; but don't demonstrate that his opinion is untenable – substantiate your own and leave it at that.

5. Be punctual and leave yourself a wide margin of time if you have to cross London to reach the College.

6. Dress neatly and soberly in a manner befitting a doctor seeking membership of a Royal College, for there are still a goodly number of examiners 'square' enough to object to patched jeans and open-necked shirts, within the confines of Princess Gate.

Finally to repeat what has been said earlier: Your examiners are General Practitioners and the vast majority of them are trying to help you; they are not trying to fail you, so be of good heart when you enter the room for your first oral. Your examiners will stand up, shake hands and introduce themselves to you and thereby set the tenor of the rest of the interview.

NOTES FOR CANDIDATES

The oral examination consists of two ½-hour orals.

The *first* oral will be devoted to questioning the candidate on his Log Diary.

Approximately one-third of the marks in this oral will be allocated to knowledge of practice organisation including the deployment of attached staff.

Although Service candidates and trainees may not have been able to influence the organisation described in their Diary, they will nevertheless be expected to have a good working knowledge of practice organisation.

The remainder of the first oral will be devoted to questioning the candidate on the management of his own cases listed in the Diary.

If the candidate has been unable to describe sufficient cases, questioning will be on the general policy of managing clinical situations in general practice, e.g. urinary tract infection, asthma, congestive cardiac failure, etc.

During the *second* oral the candidate will be questioned on the diagnosis and management of clinical problems presented by the examiners.

He may also be asked to comment on issues relating to the profession in general and general practice in particular.

Candidates will be expected to satisfy the examiners that they can apply their knowledge and skills to total personal care in clinical, psychological and social terms.

DIARY PAGE 1

THE ROYAL COLLEGE OF GENERAL PRACTITIONERS

ANALYSIS OF WORK LOAD AND PRACTICE ORGANISATION

NAME ....

ADDRESS ....

....

The following analysis will assist the Panel of Examiners to assess you in your examination performance.

The audit will not in itself attract any marks but will help the examiners to enquire into your knowledge of practice organisation and discuss with you the patients you have seen recently.

Please complete pages 1, 2 and 3 and on pages 4 and 5 record details of fifty consecutive patients seen.

1. *Practice list size*

2. *Your status in the practice—*
   Principal   Assistant   Trainee

3. *Length of experience in general practice*

4. *Number of years in post*

5. *Type of practice*
   Rural   Urban   Mixed   Dispensing
   Teaching

6. *Type of premises*
   Converted   Purpose Built   Health Centre

7. *Total number of doctors in the practice*
   (Providing General Medical Services)
   Full-time partners
   Part-time partners
   Assistants
   Trainee Assistants

8. *Obstetric commitment of the practice*
   Number of confinements in complete care
   Number of confinements in shared care
   (These figures should refer to a recent quarter for which figures are available)

9. *Total Number of night visits (11 p.m.—7 a.m.)
   made by the candidate during the most recent
   complete month*

10. **Appointments system**   YES/NO FULL/PARTIAL

11. *Special sessions: specify*   ....
       e.g. Antenatal clinic   ....
           Immunisation   ....
           Cytology   ....

12. *Staff employed: specify*   ....
    ....
    ....
    ....
    ....
    ....

13. *Staff attached: specify*   ....
    ....
    ....
    ....
    ....

14. *Additional diagnostic*   ....
       Equipment, e.g. ECG, Peak   ....
       flow meter   ....
    ....

15. *Diagnostic facilities to
    which open or direct
    access is available: specify*   ....
    ....
    ....
    ....

16. *Posts Held Outwith the Practice, e.g. hospital sessions*

....
....
....
....
....

17. *Any special characteristics of your practice to Which You wish to draw attention, e.g. teaching, geographical features, social features:*

....
....
....
....
....
....

TOTAL PRACTICE WORK LOAD OVER ONE WEEK

1. *No. of patients seen by all doctors:*

	M	Tu	W	Th	F	Sat
Consulting a.m.						
Consulting p.m.						
Other surgeries or special clinics						
New home visits						
Repeat home visits						

2. *No. of patients seen by the candidate:*

	M	Tu	W	Th	F	Sat
Consulting a.m.						
Consulting p.m.						
Other surgeries or special clinics						
New home visits						
Repeat home visits						

List consecutively *FIFTY* patients seen during the week of the audit, *in the consulting room and on home visits* (excluding special clinics)

As the examiners will wish to explore particular cases it will be in your own interest to bring an aide memoire with you.

V = Visit
S = Surgery

Date	Patient's name or initials	Age	Sex	Main reasons for contact	V	S

Date	Patient's name or initials	Age	Sex	Main reasons for contact	V	S

FIRST ORAL

You would be justified in feeling a modest sense of confidence as you confront your examiner for the first time, because this oral is based on your Log Diary. In it you have described in some detail the practice you work in, thereby giving your examiners a fairly accurate picture of the sort of doctor you think you are and, more importantly, the sort of doctor you think your examiners would like you to be!

Each section of the diary (see pages 26–31) will have been completed as accurately and honestly as possible, and it will be assumed that you not only remember what you have written but that you will have prepared yourself to be able to discuss in more detail any questions arising from the answers you have given.

After the initial courtesies have been completed some time will be spent discussing the candidate's knowledge of practice organisation and ancillary services.

Doctors who do not work in NHS practices may be in some difficulty here, but nevertheless they would be expected to have a sound grasp of practice organisation and all the personnel involved in the primary care team. About one-third of the time would be spent thus, and although few if any marks may be earned there is little doubt that the initial impression given is of the utmost importance in view of the relatively short time the examiners have to assess the candidate's expertise and personality.

Let us take the Diary page by page.

Page 1

All the questions on this page are factual and should not pose any problems. You may be asked to comment if your practice is a teaching one or your views may be sought on dispensing or the pros and cons of working from a Health Centre.

You should also have given some thought to the current arguments about home and hospital confinements – not forgetting the views of patients in the matter.

Pages 2 and 3

Section 9 You may be asked about deputising services and your criteria for the night visits.

Section 10 Be prepared to justify your attitude to appointments systems.

Section 11 Who should do the immunisations and how much, if any, of the antenatal examinations should be done by the doctor? What do you advise when your patients ask you about pertussis immunisation?

Section 12 and 13 Health Visitors, Social Workers, Practice Nurses, Receptionists and Practice Managers are always popular subjects with examiners so you should be prepared to air your views, and if you should be critical or even hostile to any one or more of these people do say so but only if you can support your stance with reasoned argument.

Section 14 Know why and how you use the equipment you have mentioned and bear in mind the caution already given about ECGs.

Section 15 What diagnostic facilities should be available to you? When, if ever, should a Consultant be interposed between you and the diagnostic facility you think you need for your patient?

The value or not of routine investigations.

The cost of such measures? When is it justified to expose your patient to possibly painful, distressing and costly procedures?

These latter sort of questions are more likely to arise in the second part of this oral or in oral 2, but they are mentioned to remind you of their increasing importance.

Section 16 A wide variety of jobs are done by doctors outside their practice and your views are likely to be sought if you are, for example, a school, factory or prison doctor or have regular hospital sessions.

Section 17 Describe the environment as best you can and don't be reticent if you really feel that you can only convey the beauty of the place by using language more flowery than is usual in such a document. Similarly if you think it is tending more to the sordid you might say so and thus open up an interesting dialogue concerning the reasons why doctors work in such places and why doctors are deserting the centres of the big cities.

Describe your patients using the Registrar General's Classification of Social Groups. Mention if there are, for example, immigrant or gipsy groups, high unemployment, good or bad Social Services and high or low crime rates in your area.

Page 4
Section 1 and 2   No great problems here, but bear in mind that the examiners are very skilled at picking out unusual features or anomalies such as – why do you see such a high (or low) proportion of the patients compared with your colleagues? Why so many (or so few) home visits and why so much more (or less) than your partners? Why so many night visits? Are you influenced by the extra payments for these? What do you think about deputising services? If you think that a doctor owes it to himself and his family to have regular and uninterrupted off-duty then say so, but argue your case as dispassionately as possible.

Special clinics might invite questions about screening, so be ready with your ideas on this controversial subject and that of say, cervical smears and paediatric developmental clinics.

Pages 5 and 6
On these pages are recorded brief notes on some fifty consecutive patients seen by you, and there is no reason why you should not edit this list somewhat, if by so doing you give it added interest by widening the range of patients seen. However they should be patients actually seen by you and you must not unbalance the average proportions of the common categories of illness seen in most practices. Too many relatively rare cases (e.g. five cases of ?myxoedema in the fifty) might arouse just a shadow of suspicion in the minds of some examiners! On the other hand if all your cases are suffering from earaches, period pains or coughs you may bore your examiner or irritate him by restricting the means whereby he can initiate a useful and revealing line of interrogation. Once again you must be ready to argue your case to support the actions you take, especially if these are at variance with majority opinion, e.g. antibiotics for diarrhoea, for earache or for non-febrile bronchitis; for sending a patient away without any treatment or with two or more therapeutic agents.

You might be asked when you think hypertension should be

treated and what your criteria are for diagnosing it?

Your opinion on the various treatments now in vogue may be sought, and it is best in this situation to know thoroughly the regimes in use in your own practice and the main contra-indications to the use of the better-known drugs. This advice applies to all drug regimes and it cannot be said too often that you should know as much as possible about treatments favoured by you for the common complaints seen in the surgery.

Have a few favourite drugs, say not less than two from each of the main groups and know their BP name, the dosage, the indications and the contraindications and if your favourite cough mixture is 'Tixylix', know the ingredients!

Know how to treat a woman with dysuria who comes to your surgery on a Friday night; know the commonest pathogen causing tonsillitis.

Support or refute the reasons for treating obesity with drugs. If you think barbiturates are of value in some situations apart from epilepsy then say so, but support your argument.

The examiners are assessing your ability to solve problems and your attitude to patients and to colleagues. They are also seeking evidence that you possess some measure of the most important attributes of all; i.e. compassion and common sense.

You need not know anything about rare syndromes and you should not be fanatical about any of the political, social or ethical dilemmas which beset us as much these days as they ever did in times past. This does not mean that you should not reveal your own code of practice or that you are expected to be prepared to compromise at all times or that you would act contrary to your own religious beliefs – a touch of eccentricity, a modicum of prejudice perhaps, often appeals to an examiner somewhat jaded by unending examples of conformity and rectitude. However, this may be a dangerous ploy if adopted deliberately by a candidate in order only to impress the examiner! Fortunately the eccentric and the strongly prejudiced amongst us are not always aware of our predilections nor of the possibility that the examiners may be similarly constituted. A most important preparation for this part of the oral is that you should carry into the examination a small notebook or aide memoire containing the details of your fifty cases. Update this before your oral so that you can give details of the outcome, results of tests and so on. (Remember your Log Diary is filled in some weeks before your actual oral so you will have more information on many cases). Do not, as some candidates have done in the past, bring all your patients case notes with you – this would be thought of as slightly odd!

6
The Problem-solving Oral

K. YOUNG

After the gong strikes, at the end of the Log Diary oral, your examiners will hand you a piece of paper on which they have briefly noted the subjects they have discussed with you. Thus your next examiners will not go over the same ground. This can be to your advantage of course; but equally well it may be to your disadvantage if in your first oral you were fortunate enough to be questioned on subjects about which you were very knowledgeable. On balance it favours the candidate since it widens the area of medical knowledge on which he may be questioned. The examiners are very unlikely to repeat any questions already covered in the MEQ and TEQ papers so this knowledge too, however minimally, is of advantage to the candidate.

This oral is essentially a problem-solving exercise and may be compared with the clinical part of your finals. You are presented with a major case and, if time allows, one or more minor cases; and once again one examiner will talk to you while the other assesses your performance.

Some examiners will hand you a slip of paper on which is recorded details of a patient and an outline of the problem to be discussed; while others may present it to you verbally.

You should read or listen to this introduction without haste and should digest every word until you are quite clear in your own mind what you are being asked. If you are not absolutely certain you must ask your examiner to elaborate. It is also quite permissible to ask for further information if you think that it is relevant to your management of the case.

Step by step the case should now unfold, rather like a MEQ except that the lines of development are much less rigid and the examiner may allow himself to play it by ear if he is satisfied that the areas you are entering are relevant to the question posed.

You might be lucky enough to detect at an early stage whether your examiner is a physically or psychosocially orientated doctor and thus be able to 'weigh' your answers accordingly. At the same time, though, you should show that you pay due heed to both attitudes, and certainly you should not disparage too vehemently either 'school' lest your marking examiner himself belongs to it!

Remember here that you should not pursue paths which may lead to areas where you are a stranger, and you should also remember that you may be able to lead your examiner into areas where you are well informed.

The examiners seek to test your common sense, your confidence and your medical expertise in everyday clinical situations, so you are unlikely to be presented with rare cases. Their assessment of your professionalism is traditionally based on your recognition, or not, of the physcial, social and psychological factors involved in a case or, more colourfully, they seek to discover if you have a 'third ear' attuned to the great variety and subtleties of human illness and the nuances of human behaviour.

In more familiar terms, the oral examination is designed 'to test the knowledge, skills and attitudes of the candidate in whole person medicine'. For the purposes of preparing for the examination this concept may be usefully considered under the following headings:

1. the recognition and solution of common problems;
2. assessment and interpretation of common physical signs and symptoms;
3. knowledge and interpretation of human behaviour;
4. communication between doctor and patient, doctor and doctor, doctor and ancillary staff, and doctor and relatives;
5. treatment and management of common emergencies;
6. knowledge of the influence of chronic disease on the individual and the community, and the effects of terminal disease and death on all those involved.

Having described at some length how you should approach each problem it would be more instructive at this point to introduce examples of the sort of questions asked (bearing in mind the limitations involved in writing about a wholly verbal transaction between an examiner and a candidate).

CASE (1)

Part 1

> Miss Good aged 53, who lives with her mother aged 83, calls to see you at your surgery and tells you she is very worried about her mother because she won't eat properly, is uncooperative and looks ill but refuses to see the doctor.

This is the way it would be put to the examinee and what follows (Part 2) may either be elicited by the candidate or offered by the examiner as the case develops.

Those parts in italics refer to the information sought by the examiner himself.

The candidate is told that he does not know the patient but does know Miss Good who saw him a year ago with ? menopausal depression – he (the doctor) had made a note that she wanted to go and housekeep for a widower friend in Scotland.

Part 2

Mother in fair condition. Ambulant. Hostile but mentally clear. You diagnose early CHF and suspect hypothyroidism, possibly hypothermia. Daughter tells you she cannot 'go on' looking after her mother.

How does he approach problem? Evaluating an elderly patient. Recognising concealed depression.

? Possibility of suicide.

? How much related to daughter's attitude and wishes.

? Diagnosis of CHF, hypothyroidism, hypothermia, etc.

Management of case in light of various possible eventualities.

CASE (2)

Part 1

> Mr Perkins, a retired chemist aged 62, is seized with a severe chest pain when weeding his garden on Sunday afternoon. He is not your patient but usually sees a local retired doctor (privately) whom he knew well in the past. His wife 'phones you and sounds very agitated and requests an urgent visit.

How does candidate react to this request.

Part 2

Case is developed and although an acute reflex oesophagitis/hiatus hernia was finally confirmed all the other possibilities were followed up in detail.

The patient is obese.

Acute myocardial infarct, ECG, hospital or home care.

The patient had concealed his dyspepsia and chest pain for some months, convinced that he had 'heart disease'.

The most severe attack came on after stooping a lot in the garden. He asks you if he can be cured by operation.

? *What does the candidate advise the patient – if not surgery how is he to cope with his disability.*

The retired doctor is very well known in the community and is a personal friend of your senior partner and the patient, unknown to you, has consulted him and has been advised that, as he is obviously suffering from 'angina' and raised blood pressure (his BP is 165/100), surgical treatment would be, at the best irrelevant, and at the worst, highly dangerous.

? *Surgical treatment or not for hiatus hernia. How does candidate manage this development and how does he deal with the retired doctor.*

If time had allowed the examiner might have asked the candidate to manage the case as if the evidence favoured a cardiac rather than an alimentary origin for the pain.

It should be noted however that either line of development allows the examiner to cover many points.

CASE (3)

Six months ago Mrs Pendry, aged 47, was admitted to the General Hospital with an 'acute abdomen' and was returned to your care with a diagnosis of carcinoma of the caecum with numerous secondaries. She does not know the diagnosis and wishes to convalesce at home.

Her husband manages his own small shop with post office.

There are two daughters aged 15 and 7, and a son aged 13.

One married sister lives in the same town, and her elderly mother lives alone two hundred miles away.

Mrs Pendry has now developed ascites; she was admitted to local GP hospital and had paracentesis of a profuse amount of fluid after which she was discharged to your care.

You might not have been given all the information mentioned above but you should elicit all the background facts that you would need to manage the case.

? What does candidate tell patient and how.

The controversial question of what the patient should be told would be examined in depth – assuming (1) that the husband agrees to her being told the truth or (2) that he does not agree, and so on.

The part the children should play would be discussed, and the pros and cons of home and hospital care for terminal illness would be reviewed.

Attitudes and approach to terminal care.
Knowledge of other supportive agencies available.
When do you use drugs, what drugs and how and when should they be given and who should give them? Finally the subject of bereavement and its management might be raised.

CASE (4)

> Your patient Charles Milden aged 32, a solicitor's clerk, has multiple sclerosis and drives to your surgery to see you. He walks quite well but uses a stick – 'for confidence' he says.
>
> He comes to tell you that he is going to marry a student teacher (also a patient of your practice) and is quite overjoyed at the prospect.
>
> She believes that he suffers from a chronic nervous condition and is very happy, because shortly after he met her he went into remission.
>
> He absolutely refuses to accept your advice that she should be told lest it jeopardize his chance of happiness.

The examiner will discuss with you at some length the natural history of MS – prognosis, treatment and its effect on the patient and his relatives.
You would be expected to pick up the fact that he was driving his car and you would be expected to know how this disease would affect his right to hold a driving licence (note too that he works in a solicitor's office).

Later his fiancée comes to see you and asks for advice on contraception. This is a very difficult question but it does demonstrate that, as with most such questions in general practice, there is no absolutely right or wrong answer. The oral examination does not therefore seek stark solutions but it does seek to elicit that your choice of action is sensible, well informed, compassionate and conforms generally to a consensus of your peers.

When the 'long' question is completed there is usually sufficient time left for the other examiner to put one or more 'short' questions to you, so you should not relax too much even if you feel that you have done well up to this point. A good performance just before the gong sounds is likely to sway the examiners more in your favour.

CASE (5)

> Mother brings along a child of 6, who has bouts of abdominal pain at any time of day. Bouts last ½ hour and she is well between attacks.
> Mother very worried about appendicitis.

The examiner would want to know what questions you would ask the mother to establish diagnosis, and expect you to be prepared to discuss a differential diagnosis which includes:

1. *emotional causes;*
2. *mesenteric adenitis;*
3. *UTI;*
4. *URTI.*

CASE (6)

> A young man aged 19 years consults you, saying he thinks he may have VD following sexual intercourse with a girl he met at a pop festival.

Find out first if he actually has a discharge, and be prepared to advise how you would manage the problem if he were:

1. *married; or*
2. *engaged to a girl with whom he has intercourse regularly.*

? What would you do if this young man had confirmed gonorrhoea and alleged that he had only had intercourse with:

1. *his wife; or*
2. *his fiancée*

CASE (7)

> You are consulted by a man aged 26 who says he is staying in the neighbourhood for 4 weeks. He says his usual GP gives him Seconal to take every night to help him sleep and he needs a further prescription.

You may wish to phone his GP and certainly you would want to know more about him.

You might be led into a short discussion on sleeping problems and their treatment. You might be asked how you treat an airline pilot who is a patient of yours who asks for sleeping tablets to help him sleep on long trips; or he may be a long-distance lorry driver, etc.

CASE (8)

A child aged 4 years whom you have not seen before has had earache for 2 hours. Temperature 38°C (R) ear drum is bulging in post/superior quadrant. Throat is red. Mucoid rhinitis. Chest clear.

? What action would you take and what treatment would you prescribe/ administer.

There would be questions about the epidemiology of upper respiratory infections in children. ? The common inrection organisms.

? The indications for using antibiotics.

? The complications ensuing from such infections.

All these examples give you some idea of what to expect in the orals. Although the younger vocationally trained doctors, as a group, tend to have a higher pass rate in the examination, older GP's should be at an advantage once the oral stage is reached. Their experience and ability to handle awkward people and situations are undoubted assets.

Chapter 9 (work plan) gives general advice about preparing for the examination, but it is worth making some points about the orals:

1. do not stop preparing once the writtens are complete; keep up with the journals and revise the general reading – especially the BNF;
2. audit your own work each day;
3. be oralled;
4. revise the contents of your emergency bag and revise your management of all the common emergencies.

If pre-oral nerves are acute then a small dose of oxyprenolol (20–40mg) half an hour beforehand can work wonders!

7
Vital Statistics

A. J. MOULDS

No-one wishes to burden their minds with a lot of useless figures. However, in many exam situations a knowledge of the approximate magnitude of a problem can be very helpful.

Many questions in the TEQ can be more fully answered by including background statistical data, while a few cannot be answered at all without the appropriate figures. The question 'Discuss whether there are too many or too few doctors in General Practice', for example, cannot be answered properly without giving approximate figures for the number of GPs, their list sizes, consultation rates, home visiting rates, emergency call rates, etc.

The Log Diary oral also needs a certain amount of statistical knowledge. You are providing an analysis of your practice and work-load and it is worth knowing how similar to, or different from, other practices you are. If you are single-handed or in a health centre or dispensing, then know how many others in the country are in the same situation. Similarly if you do no home visits or night calls or have very high consultation rates, realise that you are different and be prepared to explain why. As long as you anticipate this kind of question then marks are easily gained.

Trends in General Practice is packed full of all the information that you might need and cannot be too highly recommended.

POPULATION

Population of Great Britain	$= 55 \times 10^6$
Percentage over the age of 65	$= 15\%$ (rising)
Percentage under the age of 15	$= 20\%$
Number unemployed	$= 1.5 \times 10^6$
Life expectation, male child	$= 70$ years

Life expectation, female child   = 76 years
Births per practice per year   = 30
Deaths per practice per year   = 28–30

MEDICAL MANPOWER

Number of doctors in Great Britain = 60,000
Number of GPs in Great Britain   = 26,000
Average list size per GP   = 2,300 (Scotland
                                      1,950)
Percentage single handed   = 18%
Percentage in 2, 3, 4 man groups = 64%
Percentage in health centres   = 18%
Percentage dispensing   = 8%

WORK PATTERNS

Average time per consultation   = 6 minutes (10 if
                                      psychiatric)
Number of patients seen each day = 40-plus
Number of home visits per day   = 2–10 (very variable
                                      but all rates are
                                      declining)
Number of visits between 2300 and
    0700 hours   = 1–2 per GP per month
Percentage of patients who will
    consult at least once per year = 66%
Annual consultation rate   = 3 per patient per year
                                    = (higher in Scotland)

PRESCRIBING

Drug bill for General Practice   = £6 × 10⁸ per annum
Drug bill for individual GP   = £20,000-plus per
                                      annum
Percentage population taking
    medication on any day   = 60%
Number of prescription papers per
    patient per year   = 6.1
Percentage repeat prescriptions   = up to 50% of all
                                      prescriptions
Most commonly prescribed drugs   = Psychotropics and
                                      antibiotics

HOSPITAL

Percentage population inpatients in any year	= 11%
Percentage population new referrals to OP per year	= 15%
Percentage population self referred to A & E department per year	= 20%

8
Sources of Information

T. A. BOUCHIER HAYES

Each candidate for the MRCGP will know his own strengths and weaknesses. Those who have completed a well-constructed vocational training scheme will have been preparing for 3 years. The more mature candidate, with general practice experience, will only prepare formally for about 6 months before the examination. Their needs are different.

MEDICAL JOURNALS

Update is required reading and is an excellent source of up-to-date revision material. The previous 6 months' back numbers are necessary. The journal contains 'Clinical Challenge' which is a form of the modified essay question, with answers and discussion, and is well worth practising. For some years the Royal Australian College of General Practitioners has been producing a regular self-assessment programme in preparation for the Australian examination. Now *Update* publish their material, suitably adapted for British readers. The programmes vary considerably in their approach but all present the reader with an opportunity to review his knowledge rapidly, and to revise those aspects he wishes to cover. *Learning at Home* and the *Journal Club* are informative and worth reading. The editorials are a must for all those preparing for the examination.

Journal of the RCGP. This is worth reading, reflecting as it does current thinking on all issues related to General Practice and its research.

The British Medical Journal is now more popular and is read by many examiners. Its editorials are a source for the questions for the TEQ and form many topics for the orals (as do the editorials of the College journal).

BOOKS (a short list for the examination):

1. *British National Formulary.* Much useful information is found in the first 200 pages. It is necessary for all parts of the examination relating to drugs, their indications, actions and side-effects. There are excellent notes on guidance on prescribing, drug-dependence, drug-interaction, adverse reactions to drugs, and emergency treatment of poisoning. In my opinion *the* most important and useful book in preparation for the examination.

2. *The General Practitioner's Yearbook. An advisory guide from Winthrop.* This handsome book from Winthrop contains many items of interest to all doctors but its sections on major reports and developments, National Health Service, Acts of Parliament affecting the Medical Practitioner, Paramedical Service for the Community, etc. are essential for doctors preparing for the examination.

3. *A Textbook of Medical Practice*, Fry, J., Bryne, P. S., and Johnson, S. (MTP Press). If one textbook is appropriate, this must be the one. An everyday reference containing some delightful essays.

4. *Trends in General Practice 1977*, a collection of essays by Members of the Royal College of General Practitioners. A storehouse of facts and figures in an easily digested form.

GENERAL BOOKS

This list of books on General Practice does not claim to be comprehensive. In particular most doctors will have their own preferences for reference books on specialist clinical subjects and the clinical section simply draws attention to books that might otherwise be overlooked.

Royal College of General Practitioners (1972). *The Future General Practitioner, Learning and Teaching.* (London BMA). A source book and a discussion document. Hard work. £3.50.

Hodgkin, A. K. (1978). *Towards Earlier Diagnosis.* (Churchill Livingstone). The general chapters are worth reading. £8.50.

Fry, J. (1974). *Common Diseases, Their Nature, Incidence and Care.* (MTP Press). This book could easily have been the fifth on the short list. Highly recommended. £5.50.

Hicks, D. (1976). *Primary Health. A Review* (HMSO). A monumental review of literature on general practice to date. £9.50.

Morrell, D. C. (1976). *An Introduction to Primary Medical Care.* (Churchill Livingstone). A useful book for trainees. £1.95.

CONSULTATION

Balint, M. (1968). *The Doctor, His Patient and the Illness* (2nd edition; London: Pitman). This delightful, easily read book describes the outcome of researches by the earlier Balint Groups into the content and process of the consultation in general practice. Not for last-minute preparation, confuses more than it helps. £5.00.

Balint, M. and others (1970). *Treatment or Diagnosis.* (London: Tavistock Publications). This describes some research into repeat prescriptions. £1.25.

Balint, E. and Norell, J. S. (editors) (1973). *Six minutes for the Patient.* (Tavistock Publications). Reports on research by 'Balint Group' into the dynamics of the consultation. £2.25.

Bryne, P. S. and Long, B. E. L. (1976). *Doctors Talking to Patients.* (HMSO). An analysis of what happens in the consultation based on tape-recorded interviews between doctors and patients. £2.45.

Browne, K. and Freeling, P. (1976). *The Doctor–Patient Relationship* (2nd edition; Churchill Livingstone). A short and fascinating analysis of what happens in consultations, divided into short chapters for bedtime reading. £2.75.

CLINICAL

Watts, C. A. H. (1966). *Depressive Disorders in the Community.* (Wright). A classic work on the subject; an introduction to the management of depression in general practice. £2.75.

Illingworth, R. S. (1972). *The Normal Child. Some Problems of the First Five Years* (5th Edition; Churchill). An excellent book on behavioural problems in childhood. £6.00.

Hart, C. (Editor) (1977). *Child Care in General Practice.* (Churchill Livingstone). £5.50.

Oldershaw, K. C. (1975). *Contraception, Abortion and Sterilisation in General Practice.* First-class reference work for the surgery in a style which makes interesting reading. (Kimpton) £6.50.

Kaplan, Helen (1974). *The New Sex Therapy.* (Ballière Tindall) £8.25.

Fry, L. (1973). *Dermatology – An Illustrated Guide* (Update Publications) £5.75.

Jackson, C. R. S. (1967). *The Eye in General Practice.* (Churchill Livingstone).

Mitchell, A. R. K. (1973). *Psychological Medicine in Family Practice* (Ballière Tindall).

ORGANISATION

McKichan, N. D. (1976). *The GP and the Primary Health Care Team* (3rd Edition; Pitman). A comprehensive review of the role and work of the members of the primary health care team with useful information about organisation and administration in general practice. £6.00.

Marsh, G. and Kain-Candle, P. (1976). *Team Care in General Practice.* (Croom Helm Ltd). A description of how, through good organisation, a team may provide satisfactory care for larger numbers of patients than would generally be accepted at present. £6.95.

SOCIOLOGY

Cartwright, A (1967). *Patients and Their Doctors.* (Routledge & Kegan Paul). A sociological study of attitudes of patients to doctors and of doctors to their patients. £6.25.

RESEARCH AND EDUCATION

Weed, L. L. (1969). *Medical Records, Medical Education and Patient Care.* (Press of Cape Western Reserve University). Source book for the concept of problem-orientated medical records. £7.75.

Hart, C. R. (Editor) (1975). *Screening in General Practice.* (Churchill Livingstone). A concise yet comprehensive review of definitions, possibilities and methods. £5.00.

A General Practice Glossary. College Journal Supplement No. 3 (1973)

Medical Journals

(Frequency of publication: W – weekly; F – fortnightly; M – monthly; BM – bi-monthly; Q – quarterly)

British Medicine. 12 Kendrick Mews, Kendrick Palace, London SW7 (BM).

British Journal of Sexual Medicine. 359 Strand, London WC2R 0HP (M).

British Medical Journal. BMA Tavistock Square, London WC1H 9JR (W).

Doctor. 8 North Street, Guildford, Surrey (W).

Drug and Therapeutics Bulletin. Consumers Association, 14 Buckingham St., London WC2N 6DS (F).

General Practitioner. Haymarket Press, 5 Winsby St., London W1A 2HG (W)

Journal of the Royal College of General Practitioners. Update Publications Ltd, 33/34 Alfred Place, London WC1E 7DP (M).

Lancet. 7 Adam St, Adelphi, London WC2N 6AD (W).

Medical Digest. A. S. O'Connor, 26 Sheen Park, Richmond, Surrey (M).

Medical News. 359 Strand, London WC2R 0HP (W).

The Medical Week. Update Publications, 33–34 Alfred Place, London WC1E 7DP (W).

Medical World. 10–26 Jamestown Rd, London NW1 7DT (M).

Medicine. 7–8 Henrietta St, London WC2E 8QE (BM)

Modern Geriatrics. Empire House, 414 High Rd, Chiswick, London W4 (M).

Modern Medicine. Empire House, 414 High Rd, Chiswick, London W4 (M).

Monthly Index of Medical Specialities (MIMS). Haymarket Press, 5 Winsby St, London W1N 8AP (M).

Practice Team. Francis House, Kings Head Yard, Borough High St, London SE1 1NA (M).

Practitioner. Longman, 43–45 Annandale St, Edinburgh EH7 4AT (M).

Prescribers Journal. 6 Saint Andrews St, London EC4A 3AD (BM).

Pulse. Morgan-Grampian House, 30 Calderwood St, London SE18 6QH (W).

Update. Update Publications, 33–34 Alfred Place, London WC1E 7DP (F).

World Medicine. Clareville House, 26–27 Oxondon St, London SE1Y 4EL (F).

Papers

The past TEQ and MEQ papers without answers are available, on payment, from the Royal College of General Practitioners. There are no MCQ questions available from any source.

9
Work Plan

A. J. MOULDS

The stated aim of the MRCGP exam is to test competence. There is no arbitrary cut-off point for numbers passing, so if all candidates are up to standard then all will pass. Notwithstanding this nearly 40% will fail, so although the exam is not particularly difficult it will not be passed without a good factual grounding and preparation. Do not underestimate the work involved as very few will pass without refreshing and consolidating their knowledge.

Everyone has his own way of working and planning for his individual needs. Vocational trainees still fresh from exam battles and very much within the teaching ambit will find preparation easier than the older doctor who has often become relatively professionally isolated and is not so questioning of his own attitudes and methods of working.

The time to start is 6 months before the written exam.

A. Read the recommended journals regularly to provide a broad base of current knowledge and thought.

B. Do general reading (e.g. *Trends*/Fry's *Common Diseases*, etc.).

C. Attend local postgraduate and training meetings with GP-orientated subjects. Take every opportunity to discuss and debate, with colleagues, all aspects of General Practice.

D. Pretend an examiner is constantly with you. Question your own attitudes and methods of working. Before writing a prescription say 'Why am I giving this? What good do I think it will do?' and so on. Hopefully you will recognise and change your own bad habits before they become exposed to others!

E. Three months before the written, plan and commence an individual revision programme. Two to three hours per night for four nights a week should be ample, and rotating the subjects covered will avoid staleness. Plan to finish this programme a few days before the exam to allow everything to 'settle' in your mind.

F. If possible go on a course designed for exam candidates. This advice especially applies to older doctors, as the opportunities for argument and debate are invaluable.

G. After the writtens, get together with other candidates for discussion and mock oralling. If possible find someone with experience of the exam (an examiner would be ideal but someone who has sat the exam would also be very useful) to put you through orals.

H. Remember the College thinks in physical, psychological and social terms, and all your answers in all parts of the exam should take cognisance of this fact.

10
The Mock Examination

T. A. BOUCHIER HAYES and A. J. MOULDS

This examination contains a mock MEQ, TEQ and MCQ with their marking schedules. It is designed to give you a practice run and also as a learning experience in itself.

The best time to do this is probably about 6–8 weeks before the written examination when your level of knowledge should be reasonable, but also when there is enough time left to remedy any weaknesses exposed.

Each part must be done under examination conditions, especially as regards the timing. They could all be done on the same day; e.g.: MEQ 0930–1015; TEQ 1045–1215; MCQ 1400–1700; to give a very realistic trial or be done individually as part of your revision timetable. Whichever way you prefer, when it comes to the self-marking be fair but tough on yourself. The 'that's what I really meant so I'll give myself a mark' syndrome deludes only yourself!

After the marking re-read the appropriate chapter, the mock examination and the marking schedule all together and get all the points about technique clear in your mind.

The actual doing of the MEQ and TEQ are straightforward. The MCQ can be done either by putting T, F or D down on your own paper or by filling in the opscan sheets at the MCQ's start. This may involve some hopping about, but will familiarise you with the examination technique involved and would be the most valuable method.

NB: The answers on the opscan sheet are alternating in column, i.e.: 1, 3, 5, 7, etc. and 2, 4, 6, 8, etc. are in the same columns, so check each time that you are filling the answers in the correct space.

BEST OF LUCK!

ACKNOWLEDGEMENTS

As previously stated the MEQ has been used with the kind permission of the College. Its authors were Professors Knox and Hodgkin.

ORDER OF EXAMINATION
MEQ
TEQ
MCQ
Marking schedule MEQ
Marking schedule TEQ
Marking schedule MCQ

MEQ Mock Exam

INSTRUCTIONS

1. There are ten questions in this MEQ paper.
2. Answers should be brief and concise. Total time allowed is 45 minutes.
3. Answers should be written in the space provided; if more room is required use the reverse side of the question sheet.
4. In those questions where a definite number of answers are asked for do not give more answers than are requested (the extra answers will not be marked).
5. You are warned not to alter your answers after completing the whole MEQ and not to look through the book before you start. This may distort your natural assessment of the case and cause you to lose marks.
6. The MEQ is a test of your practical approach to a developing general practice situation. You are advised to consider what you would actually do or wish to do in the given example.
7. As a guide, an indication is given of the point at which you have completed one half of this paper.

In 1957 Mrs A., a slightly built woman aged 32, with two girls
(aged 3 and 6), moves into your area and registers with your
practice. She tells you that as a child she had rheumatism and
valvular disease of the heart. (No adequate records are available.)

1. What further four questions would you have put to the
patient to elaborate these two facts?

   1.

   2.

   3.

   4.

2. You learn that the valvular disease may have occurred at 5 years old and that she had raised blood pressure with both her pregnancies. She has reported because she is about to have a dental anaesthetic for removal of ten teeth and is afraid she might still have raised blood pressure.

On examination you find pulse regular at 90, BP 150/90, a slight displacement of the apex beat to the left. One feature of auscultation of the heart suggests that she may have mitral stenosis.

List three sounds you might have heard that would suggest this diagnosis:

1.

2.

3.

3. Enumerate four main points you would make in reply to the patient's query about her fitness for general anaesthetic and dental extraction, assuming that she has never needed digitalis.

1.

2.

3.

4.

4. The patient takes a part-time job in your surgery but does not report any illness to you or your partners until 1964 (7 years later).

Give four reasons why she may not have reported any illness to you.

1.

2.

3.

4.

5. 23.7.64—She reports that her last four periods have been heavier than normal and that her last period was 10 days ago. A vaginal examination reveals a mobile bulky uterus about the size of a 12-week gestation.

On 6.8.64 a gonadotrophin test is negative.

What three diagnoses would you consider most likely in this case and what action would you take?

1.

2.

3.

Action taken:

YOU HAVE NOW COMPLETED HALF THE MEQ.

6. If the patient had been pregnant list three problems you would need to discuss with her.

1.

2.

3.

7. In autumn 1964 the patient is found to be pregnant (EDD uncertain) and is booked for delivery in hospital. She is referred also to a physician who initially confirms your clinical cardiac findings.

While you are awaiting the physician's report, she becomes suddenly breathless with cyanosis of the lips and clinical evidence of congestive heart failure. There is no cough, chest pain or fever.

Discussion over the 'phone' with the physician reveals that he now considers the patient to be suffering not from mitral stenosis, but from a congenital atrial septal defect of the heart.

(a) If this new diagnosis of atrial septal defect is correct, describe three radiological findings in such a case.

    1.

    2.

    3.

(b) Give not more than three possible causes for the onset of cyanosis.

1.

2.

3.

8. On 27.3.65 she was delivered in hospital but went into acute heart failure just after delivery. For this reason she was not sterilised. She was kept on the Pill for 2 years until:

24.1.67 – she developed a severe continuous pain radiating down both arms especially the left. She is shocked, but there are no other fresh findings.

What are the two most likely causes of later acute incident?

1.

2.

9. On 14.2.67 on discharge from hospital, she comes to see you very angry because the hospital Physician Dr X 'has stopped her Pill'.

She says 'I was told by the Obstetricians two years ago that I must on no account stop taking the Pill and now Dr X tells me in front of the whole ward that I should never have been allowed to take the Pill; what does he know about the Pill anyway, he's a physician?'

Give two possible reasons for Mrs A's anger with Dr X.

1.

2.

How would you handle this situation?

10. Over the last 3 years Mrs A's cyanosis and symptoms of congestive failure have steadily increased. She now finds the care of her last child an increasing physical problem.

Apart from drug therapy, what steps would you take to support her?

END OF MEQ 3

TEQ Mock Exam

All three questions must be answered.

Time allowed – 90 minutes.

Q1. A man aged 55 comes to see you with anterior chest pain that is aggravated by effort, cold weather and emotion.

What is the likely diagnosis? How would you try and confirm it?

What is your plan for his management?

Q2. Give an account of the nature, quantity and costs of prescribing by general practitioners in the NHS.

How would you organise an audit of prescribing in your practice?

How would you endeavour to reduce volume and cost of your own prescribing?

Q3. You have made the diagnosis of cancer of the lung in a married woman of 66.

What arrangements do you make for terminal care?

MCQ Mock Exam

Time allowed – 3 hours.

All questions must be answered by filling in the true/false or don't know boxes on the computer marking sheets (on the three following pages).

SURNAME	INITIALS

CANDIDATE NUMBER

		0 1 2 3 4 5 6 7 8 9
	THOU.	
	HUND.	0 1 2 3 4 5 6 7 8 9
	TENS	0 1 2 3 4 5 6 7 8 9
	UNITS	0 1 2 3 4 5 6 7 8 9

PAGE No.
1

T means TRUE F means FALSE D means DO NOT KNOW

1 1A 1B 1C 1D 1E (T F D)
2 2A 2B 2C 2D 2E (T F D)
3 3A 3B 3C 3D 3E (T F D)
4 4A 4B 4C. 4D 4E (T F D)
5 5A 5B 5C 5D 5E (T F D)
6 6A 6B 6C 6D 6E (T F D)
7 7A 7B 7C 7D 7E (T F D)
8 8A 8B 8C 8D 8E (T F D)
9 9A 9B 9C 9D 9E (T F D)
10 10A 10B 10C 10D 10E (T F D)
11 11A 11B 11C 11D 11E (T F D)
12 12A 12B 12C 12D 12E (T F D)
13 13A 13B 13C 13D 13E (T F D)
14 14A 14B 14C 14D 14E (T F D)
15 15A 15B 15C 15D 15E (T F D)
16 16A 16B 16C 16D 16E (T F D)
17 17A 17B 17C 17D 17E (T F D)
18 18A 18B 18C 18D 18E (T F D)
19 19A 19B 19C 19D 19E (T F D)
20 20A 20B 20C 20D 20E (T F D)
21 21A 21B 21C 21D 21E (T F D)
22 22A 22B 22C 22D 22E (T F D)
23 23A 23B 23C 23D 23E (T F D)
24 24A 24B 24C 24D 24E (T F D)
25 25A 25B 25C 25D 25E (T F D)
26 26A 26B 26C 26D 26E (T F D)
27 27A 27B 27C 27D 27E (T F D)
28 28A 28B 28C 28D 28E (T F D)
29 29A 29B 29C 29D 29E (T F D)
30 30A 30B 30C 30D 30E (T F D)

SURNAME	INITIALS

CANDIDATE NUMBER

THOU.
| 0 1 2 3 4 5 6 7 8 9 |
| ▯ ▯ ▯ ▯ ▯ ▯ ▯ ▯ ▯ ▯ |

HUND.
| 0 1 2 3 4 5 6 7 8 9 |
| ▯ ▯ ▯ ▯ ▯ ▯ ▯ ▯ ▯ ▯ |

TENS
| 0 1 2 3 4 5 6 7 8 9 |
| ▯ ▯ ▯ ▯ ▯ ▯ ▯ ▯ ▯ ▯ |

UNITS
| 0 1 2 3 4 5 6 7 8 9 |
| ▯ ▯ ▯ ▯ ▯ ▯ ▯ ▯ ▯ ▯ |

PAGE No.
2
▯

T means TRUE F means FALSE D means DO NOT KNOW

	A	B	C	D	E
31	31A T F D	31B T F D	31C T F D	31D T F D	31E T F D
32	32A T F D	32B T F D	32C T F D	32D T F D	32E T F D
33	33A T F D	33B T F D	33C T F D	33D T F D	33E T F D
34	34A T F D	34B T F D	34C T F D	34D T F D	34E T F D
35	35A T F D	35B T F D	35C T F D	35D T F D	35E T F D
36	36A T F D	36B T F D	36C T F D	36D T F D	36E T F D
37	37A T F D	37B T F D	37C T F D	37D T F D	37E T F D
38	38A T F D	38B T F D	38C T F D	38D T F D	38E T F D
39	39A T F D	39B T F D	39C T F D	39D T F D	39E T F D
40	40A T F D	40B T F D	40C T F D	40D T F D	40E T F D
41	41A T F D	41B T F D	41C T F D	41D T F D	41E T F D
42	42A T F D	42B T F D	42C T F D	42D T F D	42E T F D
43	43A T F D	43B T F D	43C T F D	43D T F D	43E T F D
44	44A T F D	44B T F D	44C T F D	44D T F D	44E T F D
45	45A T F D	45B T F D	45C T F D	45D T F D	45E T F D
46	46A T F D	46B T F D	46C T F D	46D T F D	46E T F D
47	47A T F D	47B T F D	47C T F D	47D T F D	47E T F D
48	48A T F D	48B T F D	48C T F D	48D T F D	48E T F D
49	49A T F D	49B T F D	49C T F D	49D T F D	49E T F D
50	50A T F D	50B T F D	50C T F D	50D T F D	50E T F D
51	51A T F D	51B T F D	51C T F D	51D T F D	51E T F D
52	52A T F D	52B T F D	52C T F D	52D T F D	52E T F D
53	53A T F D	53B T F D	53C T F D	53D T F D	53E T F D
54	54A T F D	54B T F D	54C T F D	54D T F D	54E T F D
55	55A T F D	55B T F D	55C T F D	55D T F D	55E T F D
56	56A T F D	56B T F D	56C T F D	56D T F D	56E T F D
57	57A T F D	57B T F D	57C T F D	57D T F D	57E T F D
58	58A T F D	58B T F D	58C T F D	58D T F D	58E T F D
59	59A T F D	59B T F D	59C T F D	59D T F D	59E T F D
60	60A T F D	60B T F D	60C T F D	60D T F D	60E T F D

SURNAME		INITIALS

CANDIDATE NUMBER

THOU.	0 1 2 3 4 5 6 7 8 9
HUND.	0 1 2 3 4 5 6 7 8 9
	0 1 2 3 4 5 6 7 8 9
TENS	
UNITS	0 1 2 3 4 5 6 7 8 9

PAGE No.
3

T means **TRUE** F means **FALSE** D means **DO NOT KNOW**

61	61A T F D	61B T F D	61C T F D	61D T F D	61E T F D	62	62A T F D	62B T F D	62C T F D	62D T F D	62E T F D
63	63A T F D	63B T F D	63C T F D	63D T F D	63E T F D	64	64A T F D	64B T F D	64C T F D	64D T F D	64E T F D
65	65A T F D	65B T F D	65C T F D	65D T F D	65E T F D	66	66A T F D	66B T F D	66C T F D	66D T F D	66E T F D
67	67A T F D	67B T F D	67C T F D	67D T F D	67E T F D	68	68A T F D	68B T F D	68C T F D	68D T F D	68E T F D
69	69A T F D	69B T F D	69C T F D	69D T F D	69E T F D	70	70A T F D	70B T F D	70C T F D	70D T F D	70E T F D
71	71A T F D	71B T F D	71C T F D	71D T F D	71E T F D	72	72A T F D	72B T F D	72C T F D	72D T F D	72E T F D
73	73A T F D	73B T F D	73C T F D	73D T F D	73E T F D	74	74A T F D	74B T F D	74C T F D	74D T F D	74E T F D
75	75A T F D	75B T F D	75C T F D	75D T F D	75E T F D	76	76A T F D	76B T F D	76C T F D	76D T F D	76E T F D
77	77A T F D	77B T F D	77C T F D	77D T F D	77E T F D	78	78A T F D	78B T F D	78C T F D	78D T F D	78E T F D
79	79A T F D	79B T F D	79C T F D	79D T F D	79E T F D	80	80A T F D	80B T F D	80C T F D	80D T F D	80E T F D
81	81A T F D	81B T F D	81C T F D	81D T F D	81E T F D	82	82A T F D	82B T F D	82C T F D	82D T F D	82E T F D
83	83A T F D	83B T F D	83C T F D	83D T F D	83E T F D	84	84A T F D	84B T F D	84C T F D	84D T F D	84E T F D
85	85A T F D	85B T F D	85C T F D	85D T F D	85E T F D	86	86A T F D	86B T F D	86C T F D	86D T F D	86E T F D
87	87A T F D	87B T F D	87C T F D	87D T F D	87E T F D	88	88A T F D	88B T F D	88C T F D	88D T F D	88E T F D
89	89A T F D	89B T F D	89C T F D	89D T F D	89E T F D	90	90A T F D	90B T F D	90C T F D	90D T F D	90E T F D

1.(M) *Brucellosis*
- **A.** Is transmitted to man by the ingestion of infected meat.
- **B.** Presents with a persistent fever.
- **C.** May cause the spleen to become palpable.
- **D.** If chronic, may present with recurrent bouts of drenching night sweats.
- **E.** Responds to treatment with Tetracycline.

2.(T) *When prescribing hypotensive drugs it is important to remember that*
- **A.** Frusemide is a better antihypertensive than a thiadiazine.
- **B.** Beta-adrenergic blockers may precipitate cardiac failure.
- **C.** The most common adverse effect of Methyl Dopa is tiredness.
- **D.** Tricyclic antidepressants interfere with the action of many hypotensive drugs.
- **E.** Clonidine should not be stopped suddenly.

3.(Ps) *Alcoholism*
- **A.** Is due to a primary biochemical disorder.
- **B.** May present with blackouts which are transient losses of consciousness.
- **C.** May be associated with a polyneuritis.
- **D.** Has a worse prognosis in females than males.
- **E.** If treated can be followed by a gradual return to social drinking after 1 year's abstinence.

4.(O) *Oral contraceptives (combined pill)*
- **A.** Require no additional contraceptive precautions if started on the first day of the menstrual cycle.
- **B.** Should generally no longer be prescribed to women over the age of 40.
- **C.** Give a definite risk of hypertension which is greatest in the first 2 years of use.
- **D.** Give a definite risk of DVT which increases with the duration of use.
- **E.** Require regular cervical cytology because of their connection with carcinoma *in situ*.

5.(M) *Myxoedema*
  - **A.** Affects both sexes equally.
  - **B.** Is associated with pernicious anaemia.
  - **C.** May be a cause of dementia.
  - **D.** Characteristically shows exaggerated ankle jerks.
  - **E.** Should be treated with Thyroxine for a minimum of 3 years.

6.(CM) *Under the terms of the Mental Health Act 1959 compulsory admission to hospital*
  - **A.** May be to any hospital willing to receive the patient, i.e. not necessarily to a psychiatric hospital.
  - **B.** May be at the request of any relative and the Mental Welfare Officer, under Section 25.
  - **C.** If under Section 25 is for observation and the patient can be detained for 28 days.
  - **D.** Must be accompanied by medical recommendations from two doctors who have examined the patient personally, at the same time.
  - **E.** If urgent may be under Section 29 which is only effective for 3 days.

7.(Ps) *Characteristic features of bereavement may include*
  - **A.** Hostility towards others.
  - **B.** Guilt feelings.
  - **C.** An unwillingness to lead a normal life.
  - **D.** Denigration of the deceased.
  - **E.** Depression.

8.(ENT) *Deafness*
  - **A.** Can present in childhood as a behaviour problem.
  - **B.** Is most commonly caused by wax in the ear.
  - **C.** If conductive means that a tuning fork placed on the vertex is heard more loudly in the deafer ear.
  - **D.** If sensori-neural means that Rinne's test will be negative.
  - **E.** If sensori-neural may be helped by a hearing aid fitted to the better hearing ear.

9.(O) *During a normal menstrual cycle*
  - **A.** The average menstrual blood loss is 400 ml.

B. Ovulation occurs about 14 days before the onset of menstruation.

C. The basal body temperature rises after ovulation.

D. An IUCD will inhibit ovulation.

E. If premenstrual tension occurs then it is due to progesterone deficiency.

10.(M) *In Bells palsy*

A. The onset is slow and insidious.

B. The muscles of the upper and lower part of the face are affected.

C. Loss of taste sensation over the anterior 2/3 of the tongue can occur.

D. There is no loss of facial sensation.

E. If recovery is delayed then prednisolone may help.

11.(T) *In the management of angina beta-adrenergic blocking drugs act by*

A. Stimulating weight loss.

B. Inhibiting sympathetic drive to the heart.

C. Improving pulmonary ventilation.

D. Inducing diuresis.

E. Decreasing cardiac oxygen requirements during exercise.

12.(Ps) *Depression*

A. Affects single, divorced or widowed women more than married women.

B. May follow a viral infection.

C. Typically gives early morning wakening.

D. May simulate schizophrenia.

E. Can be treated by tricyclic drugs although the anti-depressant effect is not noticeable until about the tenth day.

13.(Su) *Varicose veins*

A. Are as common a cause of consultation in men as in women.

B. Are a contraindication to oral contraception.

C. Can be more fully diagnosed using the Trendelenburg test.

D. Can be treated by injection of sodium tretradecyl.

E. If treated by compression sclerotherapy will show a recurrence rate of nearly 2 out of 3 after 6 years.

14.(M) *In migraine*

A. The headache is caused by vasoconstriction of the intracranial vessels.

B. Social class 1 and 2 are most commonly affected.

C. Diagnosis is based on history not examination.

D. Attacks tend to diminish in later years.

E. Regular propranolol therapy is an effective prophylactic

15.(O) *It is correct to say that*

A. Scanty irregular periods are a contraindication to the pill.

B. A copper 7 intrauterine device should be changed every 18 months.

C. A diaphragm with chemicals is as effective a contraceptive as a coil.

D. The rhythm method is not as effective contraceptively as coitus interruptus.

E. Vasectomy can lead to impotence.

16.(Ps) *Characteristic features of endogenous depression include*

A. Improvement of mood in the evening.

B. Feelings of guilt.

C. Clouding of consciousness.

D. Fatigue.

E. Failure to recognise the need for treatment.

17.(D) *In acne vulgaris*

A. The primary defect appears to be excess keratin production preventing escape of sebum.

B. Males are more commonly affected than females.

C. Teenagers in the south of England have less severe acne than in the north.

D. Tetracycline therapy is often beneficial.

E. Keeping the face clean with plenty of soap and water should be recommended.

18.(M) *Ankylosing spondylitis*
  A. Seldom starts before the age of 30.
  B. Has a strong tendency to be familial.
  C. May present as sciatica.
  D. May be complicated by aortic valvular lesions.
  E. Is best treated by radiotherapy.

19.(CM) *An age–sex register may be used*
  A. To keep a record of patients suffering from specific diseases.
  B. To obtain controls for research purposes.
  C. To monitor repeat prescriptions.
  D. For assembling groups of patients for screening for specific diseases.
  E. To provide a statistical breakdown of the practice population.

20.(Ps) *In patients suffering from hysteria*
  A. The onset of symptoms is usually gradual.
  B. There is abnormal suggestibility.
  C. Hallucinations can occur.
  D. Numbness would follow a segmental or peripheral nerve distribution.
  E. There is conscious awareness that symptoms have been initiated for some personal gain.

21.(Pa) *In the development of an infant*
  A. A study of his behaviour and reactions to standard stimuli from 1 month onwards will give his Development Quotient or DQ.
  B. Intelligence Quotient or IQ cannot be measured until the age of 3 years.
  C. Stimulation from outside sources will have an accelerating effect.
  D. Severe retardation in any single field suggests mental retardation.
  E. The rate of development is constant.

22.(M) *In obesity*
  A. By far the commonest aetiological factor is overeating.

B. Life expectation is reduced in direct proportion to the degree of obesity.

C. Right ventricular failure may develop.

D. Insulin resistance may develop.

E. Group therapy can be very effective.

23.(O) *Fibroids of the uterus*

A. Occur in nearly one-third of women over the age of 40.

B. Are commoner in Negresses.

C. Characteristically present with an altered menstrual cycle.

D. If small and symptomless require no treatment.

E. Can be treated by curettage.

24.(Ps) *Aggressive psychopaths show*

A. An inability to profit from experience.

B. A tendency to premeditated violence.

C. Undue guilt and remorse after their transgressions.

D. An abnormal EEG in 2 out of 3 cases.

E. A poor response to all forms of treatment.

25.(Pa) *With normal development an infant should be able to*

A. Smile at 2 months.

B. Sit momentarily without support at 6 months.

C. Grasp with finger and thumb at 9 months.

D. Recognise its own name by 14 months.

E. Walk up and down stairs at 18 months.

26.(M) *In iron deficiency anaemia*

A. The MCHC will be above 32G per cent.

B. The most important cause is haemorrhage.

C. Koilonychia is characteristic.

D. The patient may complain of a sore tongue.

E. The iron and iron-binding levels in the plasma are lowered.

27.(T) *Synthetic corticosteroids by mouth may cause*

A. Osteoporosis.

B. Depression with risk of suicide.

C. Peptic ulceration.

D. Venous thrombosis.

E. Delayed wound healing.

28.(Su) *Torsion of the testicle*

A. Occurs most commonly in teenagers.

B. May be misdiagnosed as orchitis.

C. Should be treated as an emergency.

D. Occurs more commonly in undescended testicles.

E. Should be reduced by manipulation before referral to hospital.

29.(Pa) *Compared to cow's milk, breast milk*

A. Has less calories.

B. Has less protein.

C. Has less iron.

D. Has more sodium.

E. Is less likely to cause tetany.

30.(M) *A married 50-year-old postman has made an uncomplicated recovery from a first myocardial infarction. He should be advised to*

A. Give up his job and retire early.

B. Never smoke again.

C. Go onto a high fibre diet.

D. Have an ECG every 6 months.

E. Refrain from sexual intercourse for 1 year after the episode.

31.(Op) *In young children who squint it is correct to say that*

A. They are nearly all long-sighted.

B. The cover test is of little diagnostic value.

C. Amblyopia (lazy eye) is rarely improved by treatment after the age of 7.

D. Concomitant squint should be treated by occluding the master eye and so forcing the child to use the squinting eye.

E. Orthoptic exercises are designed to strengthen the eye muscles.

32.(Ps) *Characteristic features of schizophrenia include*

A. Clouding of consciousness.
B. Impaired memory.
C. Apathy and indifference.
D. A feeling of being under the influence of an external force.
E. A feeling of being the centre of the whole world.

33.(O) *At the menopause*
A. Menstruation most commonly ceases at 45–46.
B. The serum cholesterol is reduced.
C. Vasomotor instability is characteristic.
D. Bleeding after 1 year's amenorrhoea requires further investigation.
E. Hormone replacement therapy may well be associated with an increased risk of endometrial cancer.

34.(M) *In peptic ulceration*
A. Gastric ulcers affect both sexes almost equally.
B. Duodenal ulcers are evenly distributed throughout the social classes.
C. Gastric ulcers are associated with normal or slightly raised gastric acidity.
D. If a gastric ulcer is not on the lesser curvature then there is a greater risk of it's being malignant.
E. Duodenal ulcer typically causes hunger pains.

35.(Pa) *Breast feeding*
A. Gives the mother significant protection against carcinoma of the breast.
B. Protects the baby from cot death.
C. Has a contraceptive effect.
D. Decreases the risk of the baby developing eczema.
E. Requires supplementing with Vitamin C after 6 weeks.

36.(Ps) *Recognised features of anorexia nervosa are*
A. Menorrhagia.
B. Lethargy.
C. A distorted concept of body image.
D. 'Belle indifference'.
E. Hypokalaemia.

37.(Op) *Painful red eye*
- **A.** Associated with keratic precipitates is characteristic of acute iritis.
- **B.** Associated with inactive semi-dilated pupil is characteristic of acute keratitis.
- **C.** Associated with a generalised conjunctival infection is characteristic of acute conjunctivitis.
- **D.** Caused by acute iritis should be treated with as much topical corticosteroid as is needed to keep the eye quiet.
- **E.** Caused by acute glaucoma should be treated with mydriatics.

38.(M) *A patient with*
- **A.** Epilepsy is not allowed to drive until 2 years without a fit.
- **B.** Pernicious anaemia may have subacute combined degeneration of the cord precipitated by folic acid therapy.
- **C.** Angina may have no evidence of myocardial ischaemia on ECG.
- **D.** An MSSU showing 10^4 organisms per ml has an acute urinary tract infection.
- **E.** Asthma can have the severity of his attack determined by a chest x-ray.

39.(Ps) *Recognised side-effects of amitryptilline are*
- **A.** Diarrhoea.
- **B.** Heart block.
- **C.** Weight gain.
- **D.** Anxiety.
- **E.** Precipitation of glaucoma.

40.(ENT) *Ménières disease (Labyrinthine vertigo)*
- **A.** Affects women more often than men.
- **B.** Is a disease of middle age.
- **C.** May give a loss of consciousness during an acute attack.
- **D.** Is differentiated from lesions of the auditory nerve by the recruitment test.
- **E.** Can be treated routinely with prochlorperazine (Stemetil) 10 mg oral t.i.d.

41.(CM) *It is correct to say that*
- **A.** Up to 50% of consultations in general practice do not lead to a precise diagnosis.
- **B.** Three out of 4 symptoms are treated in the community without medical advice or assistance.
- **C.** Emotional disorders are the commonest group of minor conditions dealt with by the GP.
- **D.** About one doctor per month commits suicide.
- **E.** Two out of three children (below the age of 10) will be seen each year, by their GP, with a respiratory disorder.

42.(M) *In thyrotoxicosis*
- **A.** The hands are warm and moist with a coarse tremor.
- **B.** Dermatographia is a feature.
- **C.** The ECG may show atrial flutter.
- **D.** Exophthalmos may not respond to the treatment of the thyroid overactivity.
- **E.** After successful treatment with radioactive iodine, long-term follow up is not indicated.

43.(T) *In an acute asthmatic attack in a 15-year-old boy*
- **A.** Disodium cromoglycate (Intal) is effective and free from side-effects.
- **B.** Intravenous aminophylline should be given at a rate not exceeding 2 ml per minute.
- **C.** Doubling the dose of his steroid aerosol will help.
- **D.** Parenteral hydrocortisone should be reserved for hospital administration.
- **E.** Salbutamol may give cardiac toxicity if he is hypoxic.

44.(O) *Monilial vaginitis*
- **A.** Is caused by a fungus which prefers an acid medium for growth.
- **B.** Shows an increased incidence in pregnancy.
- **C.** Causes intense pruritis.
- **D.** May follow treatment with a broad-spectrum antibiotic.
- **E.** Can present with a watery or purulent discharge.

45.(Su) *Carcinoma of the breast*
- **A.** Causes about 20% of all deaths from malignant disease

in the UK.
- **B.** Is more likely to occur in a nulliparous woman.
- **C.** Is always an adenocarcinoma.
- **D.** Generally presents with the patient complaining of discomfort or pain in the breast.
- **E.** Should be treated with simple mastectomy as there is no evidence that more radical operations give improved survival rates.

46.(M) *In hiatus hernia*
- **A.** Symptoms are caused by reflux oesophagitis.
- **B.** The substernal pain may be brought on by exercise.
- **C.** Anaemia may be the presenting feature.
- **D.** Sleeping with the foot of the bed raised often helps.
- **E.** Reduction of weight helps to relieve symptoms.

47.(Ps) *The autistic child*
- **A.** Is interested in things not people.
- **B.** Has a tendency to self-injury.
- **C.** Generally has a gross speech disturbance.
- **D.** Shows an obsessive need to change his environment.
- **E.** May show frank manifestations of schizophrenia in adolescence.

48.(Pa) *Threadworm infestation*
- **A.** Is often asymptomatic.
- **B.** If chronic can cause iron deficiency anaemia.
- **C.** May provoke pneumonitis.
- **D.** Generally affects the other children in a family but rarely the adults.
- **E.** Can be easily treated by a single dose of piperazine sulphate and standardised senna.

49.(O) *In ectopic pregnancy*
- **A.** The most important aetiological factor is previous pelvic inflammatory disease.
- **B.** Bleeding is the first symptom followed by pain.
- **C.** Shoulder-tip pain may be present.
- **D.** Diagnosis rests on clinical history and not on physical signs.
- **E.** A positive gravindex aids the diagnosis.

50.(M) *Finger clubbing is a recognised feature of*
  A. Sarcoidosis.
  B. Subacute bacterial endocarditis.
  C. Chronic bronchitis.
  D. Carcinoma of the bronchus.
  E. Staphylococcal pneumonia.

51.(Ps) *The risk of suicide is*
  A. Greater in the unemployed.
  B. Unaffected by a previous attempt.
  C. Decreased in times of war.
  D. Positively associated with a recent visit to a GP.
  E. Falling in Britain as measured by mortality.

52.(CM) *In immunisation procedures*
  A. There should be at least a 3-week interval between small-pox vaccination and yellow fever vaccination, no matter which is given first.
  B. If a severe febrile reaction occurs with the first dose of triple vaccine then it is safe to give a second dose of diphtheria and tetanus vaccine.
  C. Pregnancy should be avoided for at least 9 months after rubella vaccination.
  D. BCG is indicated in tuberculin-positive children.
  E. An international certificate for primary cholera vaccination becomes valid after 2 days.

53.(T) *The thiadiazine diuretics*
  A. Increase potassium excretion.
  B. Increase sodium excretion.
  C. Increase uric acid excretion.
  D. May produce a diabetic state.
  E. Act for about 6 hours.

54.(M) *In haemophilia*
  A. Only about two-thirds of cases have a family history of the disorder.
  B. All the sons of a haemophiliac would be unaffected.
  C. All the daughters of a carrier would be carriers themselves.
  D. The deficiency is one of Factor 9.

E. Cryoprecipitate enables the anti-haemophilic globulin from a pint of plasma to be given in a 20 ml injection.

55.(Ps) *Neurotic behaviour is characterised by*
  A. A disturbed conception of reality.
  B. Complaints for which no organic cause can be found.
  C. Denial of the need for help.
  D. Malingering.
  E. Feelings of panic.

56.(O) *The following drugs may affect the development of the fetus*
  A. Aspirin.
  B. Phenobarbitone.
  C. Carbimazole.
  D. Paracetamol.
  E. Progestogens.

57.(Pa) *In non-accidental injury to children*
  A. The child may be brought some time after the injury for treatment.
  B. A spiral fracture of a limb would be virtually diagnostic.
  C. The parents are always social class 4 or 5.
  D. Once the parents know they are suspected and under supervision the child is safe from further harm.
  E. A skeletal survey should be done.

58.(M) *In diabetes mellitus*
  A. There are as many undetected diabetics as there are known cases.
  B. Cortisone therapy reduces insulin requirements.
  C. A patient on soluble insulin 80 strength drawn up to 4 marks on the syringe is injecting 20 units.
  D. Soluble insulin and PZl can be given in the same syringe.
  E. If the patient has gastroenteritis then the insulin should be reduced until normal appetite returns.

59.(Op) *Simple glaucoma*
  A. Is rare before middle age.
  B. Occurs especially in myopes.
  C. Is responsible for nearly 15% of blindness in the UK.

D. Is a cause of optic atrophy.

E. Can be treated with pilocarpine drops 1–4%.

60.(T) *The following may predispose a patient to digoxin toxicity*

A. Renal insufficiency.

B. A raised serum potassium.

C. Recent digoxin therapy.

D. Old age.

E. A low cardiac output.

61.(D) *Pityriasis rosea*

A. Mainly occurs in the over 40s.

B. Is characterised by an initial solitary lesion which may remain the only sign for up to 4 weeks before the generalised rash appears.

C. Is generally confined to the 'vest and pants' area.

D. Is a psychosomatic illness.

E. Will clear within 1 month of the onset of the generalised rash.

62.(M) *Disseminated sclerosis*

A. Shows an increased incidence with distance from the equator.

B. Is commoner in social classes 4 and 5.

C. Characteristically can present with retrobulbar neuritis.

D. Causes spastic weakness of the limbs.

E. In about one-third of patients is associated with euphoria.

63.(Ps) *In primary senile dementia*

A. Remote memory is lost before recent memory.

B. Disorientation can affect all spheres.

C. Emotional lability is characteristic.

D. Paranoia inevitably develops.

E. Vigorous and enthusiastic treatment can halt the disease process.

64(O) *Premature labour is associated with*

A. Hydramnios.

B. Neonatal death.

C. Twins.

D. Pulmonary TB.

E. Haemolytic disease of the newborn.

65.(Pa) *Congenital pyloric stenosis*
  A. Affects males and females equally.
  B. Causes symptoms when the baby first takes solid food.
  C. Characteristically causes constipation and a reluctance to feed.
  D. If suspected may best be confirmed after a test feed.
  E. Should be treated surgically with the Fredet–Ramstedt operation.

66.(M) *The carpal tunnel syndrome is*
  A. Caused by compression of the median nerve.
  B. A possible complication of pregnancy.
  C. Associated with paraesthesia of the little and ring finger.
  D. Worsened by manual work.
  E. Characteristically more painful at night.

67.(Ps) *Dementia may be caused by*
  A. Lead poisoning.
  B. Cushing's disease.
  C. Aseptic meningitis.
  D. Brain neoplasm.
  E. Huntington's chorea.

68.(Su) *It is correct to say that*
  A. In carcinoma of the distal colon increasing constipation is usually the first symptom.
  B. The usual type of anaemia post-gastrectomy is megaloblastic.
  C. A past history of piles often delays the diagnosis of carcinoma of the rectum.
  D. Diverticulosis should be treated with a low roughage diet and faecal softeners.
  E. Pale stools and urobilinogen in the urine are characteristic of obstructive jaundice.

69.(Pa) *The neonatal apgar score is based on*
  A. Fontanelle pressure.
  B. Heart rate.

C. Pupil reaction to light.
D. Colour.
E. Respiratory effort.

70.(M) *In a 50-year-old man with a BP of 180/115 on three separate recordings*
A. Right ventricular hypertrophy may be present.
B. Arteriovenous nipping would suggest the hypertension is not of recent onset.
C. An IVP would be an appropriate first line investigation.
D. The aim of therapy is to get his BP to 120/80.
E. Guanethidine may lead to failure of ejaculation.

71.(D) *Psoriasis*
A. Affects nearly 2% of the population of the UK.
B. In half of acute cases is caused by a delayed allergic reaction to a beta-haemolytic streptococcal throat infection.
C. Rarely involves the nails.
D. Is often greatly helped by a course of UV light (in sub-erythema doses).
E. Is one condition where oral corticosteroids have virtually no place in the management.

72.(T) *A patient who has ingested 20 grammes of paracetamol*
A. May look and feel well initially.
B. Is likely to develop indigestion.
C. Should have plasma paracetamol levels monitored.
D. May be treated at home after administration of emetics.
E. May develop severe hepatic failure without developing jaundice.

73.(ENT) *Acute otitis media in children*
A. Is caused by bacteria in over 90% of cases.
B. Is a recurrent condition.
C. Can be treated with tetracycline syrup.
D. Does not require follow-up.
E. Does not lead to persistent deafness.

74.(M) *In a patient with*

A. An URTI and yellow nasal discharge, an antibiotic will substantially shorten the period of infection.
B. Asthma, the peak flow meter provides a useful guide to the severity of airways obstruction.
C. Hay fever, skin testing for allergies should always be done.
D. Chronic bronchitis, breath sounds are vesicular with prolonged inspiration.
E. Asbestosis, carcinoma of the bronchus is a common complication.

75.(Ps) *In psychiatric symptomatology*
A. Neologisms are a flow of unconnected words.
B. Formication describes a form of creeping sensation under the skin.
C. Perseveration is the repetition of a recent action in spite of the patient's effort to produce a new action.
D. Illusions are mental impressions of sensory vividness occurring without external stimulus.
E. Echolalia is the repetition of words heard.

76.(O) *The following may cause breech presentation*
A. Prematurity.
B. Any condition preventing engagement of the head in the pelvis.
C. Obesity.
D. Extended legs.
E. Multiple pregnancy.

77.(Pa) *In childhood infectious disease it is correct to say that*
A. In measles the fever subsides when the rash first appears.
B. In chickenpox the skin rash is most profuse at the periphery and sparsest on the trunk.
C. The incubation period of whooping cough is 10–14 days.
D. The rash in rubella appears on the third day.
E. Petechial spots on the soft palate are a characteristic feature of measles.

78.(T) *When prescribing for the elderly the doctor should*
A. Keep drug schedules as simple as possible.
B. Always start with the standard adult dose and lower it if

side-effects develop.

C. Avoid high doses of chlorpromazine (Largactil) as it may provoke hypothermia.

D. Treat every symptom that may develop to maintain the patient's level of health.

E. Be aware that unwanted side-effects are more common.

79.(CM) *The Registrar General's social classification*

A. Is based on the present or past occupation of the head of the family.

B. Allows individuals to change class if their income alters substantially.

C. Divides the population into six major classes.

D. Provides valuable information about the association between disease and social circumstances.

E. Puts GPs and consultants into Class 1 but Junior hospital doctors into Class 2.

80.(Pa) *It is correct to say that*

A. Nocturnal enuresis with daytime control in a 6-year-old should be investigated by a micturating cystogram.

B. Febrile non-renal conditions in children can cause proteinuria.

C. Paracetamol syrup is a suitable analgesic and sedative for an infant with a cold.

D. Intussusception is a common cause of acute abdominal pain in infants.

E. Secondary nocturnal enuresis generally has a psychological cause.

81.(Ps) *Psychosexually it is correct to say that*

A. Men are at the peak of their sexual responsiveness and capacity at age 17–18.

B. Masturbation is a normal stage of sexual development.

C. Exhibitionism has the highest rate of recidivism among sexual offenders.

D. Female homosexual behaviour is an offence under the Sexual Offences Act 1967 unless in private between consenting adults.

E. Premature ejaculation is not readily amenable to treatment.

82.(M) *Leukaemia*
  A. Occurs mainly in children.
  B. Is commoner in Down's syndrome.
  C. May present with pruritis.
  D. If chronic myeloid may have painful priapism as an early symptom.
  E. If acute then in the early stages may be mistaken for aplastic anaemia.

83.(O) *Abortion*
  A. Generally presents as bleeding followed by pain.
  B. Before 12 weeks is, in the majority of cases, due to chromosomal abnormality.
  C. If threatened and followed by pregnancy to term then is not associated with an increased risk to the fetus.
  D. If recurrent (more than three times) before 12–14 weeks implies cervical incompetence.
  E. May be followed by choriocarcinoma.

84.(T) *In the drug treatment of rheumatoid arthritis*
  A. Paracetamol has only a mild anti-inflammatory effect.
  B. Pain may be temporarily increased if indomethacin is suddenly stopped.
  C. Chloroquine is safe provided the retinae are checked every 3 months.
  D. Gold salts give immediate benefit.
  E. Phenylbutazone should not be given if there is a past history of peptic ulceration.

85.(D) *Erythema nodosum may be caused by*
  A. Systemic lupus erythematosus.

B. Sarcoidosis.

C. Herpes simplex infections.

D. Primary tuberculous infection.

E. Delayed allergic response to beta-haemolytic strepto-coccal throat infections.

86.(Ps) *Schizophrenic patients*

A. Generally present in the early 30s.

B. Rarely have a family history of the disease.

C. Form the majority of long-term mental hospital patients.

D. Get feelings of panic when shopping.

E. Recover better if the onset is acute.

87.(Su) *The following disorders, in time, may give rise to malignant change*

A. Chronic duodenal ulcer.

B. Ulcerative colitis.

C. Papilloma of the bladder.

D. Diverticulitis

E. Senile keratosis.

88.(O) *During the antenatal period*

A. Hypertension, albuminuria and oedema at 14 weeks would be diagnosed as PET.

B. All patients should have a chest x-ray to exclude TB.

C. Cervical cytology is associated with a greater number of false positives.

D. Vaginal examination and assessment should be carried out at 36 weeks.

E. The head should be engaged by 39 weeks in the parous patient.

89.(T) *The following are recognised side-effects of the drugs named*

A. Maculopapular rash in more than a third of patients with ampicillin.

B. Aplastic anaemia with chloramphenicol.

C. 8th cranial nerve damage with streptomycin.
D. Exacerbation of renal failure with tetracycline.
E. Jaundice with erythromycin.

90.(Ps) *In psychiatric therapy*
A. ECT can help where amnesia is present.
B. Diazepam (Valium) can release latent aggression.
C. Chlorpromazine (Largactil) can cause obstructive jaundice.
D. ECT is of value in the treatment of manic states.
E. Haloperidol is effective in controlling psychotic excitement.

Answers to Mock MEQ

Total
possible

1. *Marks for only three of the possible answers:*

   1. Any questions that elaborated cardiac function and effect of valvular disease, dyspnoea, oedema, chest pain, etc.   4

   2. Any relation of cardiac function to pregnancy   6

   3. Queries developing an assessment of severity of original attack (attacks)
Repeated attacks
Length of time in bed or in hospital
Previous treatment, etc.   2
ALLOWED: dates of attacks of rheumatism and how treated.
Was surgery/valvotomy considered?

Total possible   —
12

NOT ALLOWED:
for Answer 1. Has she any symptoms now?
            (Nature of symptoms not given)
            Any residual disability?
            (Nature not specified)
for Answer 3. 'What valve disease and when?'

2. Any three sounds heard given three marks:
Pre-systolic murmur   3

	Total possible
Diastolic murmur	3
Accentuated second sound. Pulmonary	3
Opening snap	3
Third heart sound/Split second sound/Pulmonary area	3
Accentuated 1st sound (mitral or apex)	3
Apical systolic murmur of mitral incompetence	3
Split mitral 2nd sound	3

Total possible   9

NOT ALLOWED:
Murmurs timing not specified
A diastolic murmur over aortic area
A loud aortic 2nd sound
Systolic murmur site unspecified
Diastolic + radiation to axilla
High pitch 2nd sound at apex
Accentuated apical 2nd sound
Diastolic thrill in mitral area
A closing snap after 2nd sound

3. This question to be marked on only two of the possible answers:

1. She must have course of antibiotics   4

2. You may have to raise the question of hospital or at least a competent anaesthetist with dentist. No general anaesthetic in dental surgery   3
Doctor must inform the dentist of her history of rheumatic fever and valvular heart disease

Total possible   7

NOT ALLOWED:
She might need a prophylactic cover of antibiotic
In consultation with dental surgeon, depending on

Total
possible

severity of heart condition and general health, I
might advise operation to be carried out in two or
more stages

That she should inform the dentist or anaesthetist of
the facts (letter from General Practitioner would be
helpful).

4. *Any four of the following gain marks:*

   1. May not have had any symptoms or she has been
      too busy to notice them

   2. She may tend to minimise her disability because:
      – mothers and cardiac patients often do
      – doctors appear to be too busy
      – she is chronically ill
      – of the insidious onset
      – of fear of neurosis
      – comparison with other patients reassures her   1

   3. Difficulty on adjusting to dual role of employer/
      doctor   1

   4. May have gone privately elsewhere – not been
      our patient   1

   5. Afraid to mention symptoms because afraid severe
      illness will stop her working
      – needs money
      – loves job
      – operation or hospital   1

   6. May expect doctors to notice her symptoms auto-
      matically   1

   7. Reluctance because other staff have access to her
      records   1

                                  Total possible   4

Total
possible

5. (a) *Any three of the following:*
  Fibroids   3
  Pregnancy with false negative test (with or with-
  out mention of threatened or incomplete abor-
  tion)   4
  Dysfunctional uterine bleeding/metropathia 3
  Missed abortion (carneous mole)   3
  Endometriosis   1
  Carcinoma of body of uterus – uterine tumour 1
 NOT ALLOWED: Menorrhagia (unqualified)

(b) *What action would you take?*
  Action taken – any of the following:
  – referral to obstetrician, cardiologist or physician
  – second opinion
  – probably dilation and currettage   3
  – repeat pregnancy test

            —
        Total possible 13

NOT ALLOWED:
Ovarian tumour chorionepithelioma menorrhagia,
Endometrial polyp, endometritis, menopausal bleeding

6. *Any three of the following:*
 – confinement must be in a Specialist Unit under a
  cardiologist in hospital   3
 – hospital confinement with sterilisation after delivery   3
 – hospital confinement with subsequent adequate
  contraceptive advice
 – termination, or possibility of it   3
 – hazards of continuing pregnancy justify therapeutic abortion on medical grounds   3

Total
possible

– the need to obtain adequate rest during this pregnancy   3
– adequate care of the family (by Welfare Services, etc.)   3

———

Total possible   9

Note : Candidates lost out if they mention other 'problems' as opposed to the 'courses of action' intended.

7. (a) *Any three of the following :*

enlarged right side of heart   2
enlarged right auricle or atrium
dilated pulmonary arteries or enlarged hilar shadows   2
hilar dance   2
pulmonary congestion or increased vascular markings   2
enlarged heart   1
small aortic knuckle   2

NOT ALLOWED – Left ventricular enlargement, right ventricular enlargement.

(b) *Any three of the following :*

reversal of shunt (right to left)   2
multiple minute pulmonary emboli or infarcts; pulmonary thrombosis   1
endocarditis; subacute endocarditis has supervened   1
congestive heart failure/decompensation pulmonary oedema   1
intercurrent chest infection   1

———

Total possible   10

NOT ALLOWED – Pneumothorax or onset of atrial fibrillation, peripheral stasis, myocardial infarct.

*Total
possible*

8. *Any two of the following:*
    pulmonary infarct or embolus   3
    myocardial infarct or coronary thrombosis
    coronary insufficiency or oedema   2
    thrombosis of veins of both upper extremities
    (thrombo-embolism)   1
    thrombosis in pulmonary vessels   2
                                                                   ———
                                    Total possible   5

NOT ALLOWED – Myocarditis

9. (a) *Only two of the possible answers to be awarded marks.*
        private matters were felt to have been made
        public   3
        she had always been frightened by Pill and now
        discovers she was right
        or – Insecurity because the Pill has been stopped,
        with fear of pregnancy or altered marriage
        relationship   2

What would you say to Mrs A?

(b) *All of the following:*
        accept the anger by understanding attitude   1
        explain reasons for physician's statement   1
        confirm that Dr X is right and Pill should be
        stopped now with or without discussion of other
        birth-control methods   1
                                                                   ———
                                    Total possible   8

NOT ALLOWED: 'Reassure'.

Total possible

10. *All of the following:*

    1. Entry to nurseries or nursery schools, play group, early school entry or other help with schooling of children   1

    2. Home help service   1

    3. Meals on wheels (or local authority laundry service)   1

    4. Neighbours or relatives (including husband and daughters) help. Baby minders   1

    5. Transport to and from school   1

    6. Discuss with children's department, i.e. Children's Officer or School Medical Officer   1

    7. Housing: downstairs bedroom or bungalow; essential needs on a single floor   1

    8. Health Visitor (or District Nurse, or Social Worker)   1

    9. Stop her doing part-time work. Refer to Social Security if financial difficulties   1

                                                Total possible   9

NO MARKS FOR: Convalescent home for short spell Holidays for children.

Answers to Mock TEQ

EXAMPLES
Question 1

A man aged 55 comes to see you with anterior chest pain that is aggravated by effort, cold weather and emotion.

What is the likely diagnosis? How would you try and confirm it?

What is your plan for his management?

(*Background:* There has been much progress and discussion in care of angina over the past few years, i.e. beta-blockers, lipids, coronary artery bypass surgery, relation to high blood pressure, preventive measures. Consider how you might refer to these trends. If possible try and show that you have read about these advances.)

Answer
Likely diagnosis

The most likely diagnosis must be angina – develop this by stating the site, type, radiation, triggers of the pain	0.5 marks
Consider other possible causes such as hiatus hernia, anxiety state and anything else you want to put forward	0.5 marks

Confirmation

ECG – what use and what limitations? – note exercise ECG	1 mark
The practical value of the therapeutic test of trinitrin	0.5 marks

Plan for management

Here you should refer to the likely natural history

107

and prognosis of angina in a man of 55 and note risk
factors such as FH, high blood lipids (and which
ones), raised BP, obesity, smoking, lack of exercise
and way of life   1 mark
Then set out your plan:

1. Education and information for the patient, i.e.
   explain what he is suffering from and how he can
   help himself and what you can do for him.   1 mark

2. Preventive measures, i.e. weight control, smoking, diet, lipids, exercise, personal problems.   1 mark

3. Plan for regular follow-up. How do you assess
   progress in general practice? What do you
   check? History, TNT consumption, BP, lipids,
   exercise tolerance, etc. How often do you see
   him?   1 mark

4. Medication
     what and why and when?
     TNT?
     beta-blockers?
     diuretics
     clofibrate?
     anti-hypertensives?   1.5 marks

5. Surgery
     limitation of availability of coronary artery
     by-pass operation
     refer to reviews or papers
     the situations in USA and UK
     what indications?
     what results?
     what plans for this patient?   0.5 marks

6. Referral to cardiologist. What would be indications for referral?   0.5 marks

7. Family. Arrangements to be made to see wife to discuss his care.   0.5 marks

8. Conclusions and summary. Give 5–6 lines on the main points you have made.   0.5 marks

Question 2

Give an account of the nature, quantity and costs of prescribing by general practitioners in the NHS.

How would you organise an audit of prescribing in your practice?

How would you endeavour to reduce volume and cost of your own prescribing?

(*Background:* Highly topical on the need to control costs of NHS and to try and improve quality of prescribing.)

Subject reviewed in *Trends 1977* by Supplement to *Journal of RCGP* by Parish 1976 and editorials in this journal and in *Update*).

There are three distinct points to this question:

1. Facts on prescribing in NHS – you may not know them but have a go!

2. Audit of your practice.

3. Your own habits.

Answer

1. Facts. Over 300 million scripts per year in NHS, i.e. over 6 scripts per person per year   0.5 marks

    Volume increasing annually   0.5 marks

    Costs now about £569 million per year for GP NHS prescriptions   0.5 marks

    Over £1.50 per script   0.5 marks

Prescribing cost per GP per year (1977) was around £20,000 per GP   0.5 marks

Content. Largest groups:

For respiratory disorders:
    CVS
    psychotropic drugs
    analgesics
    alimentary system
    skin
    anti-rheumatic   1 mark

2. Audit
    how would you record practice prescribing?
    how would you organise practice group dis-
    cussions?
    how would you monitor costs?
    how would you influence changes?   2 marks

3. Own prescribing
    More detailed analysis of your own prescrib-
    ing?
    what would you question and how would you
    check?
    i.e. about – antibiotics; anti-hypertensives;
    anti-rheumatics
    how might you organise controlled trials for
    efficacy?
    How would you measure effects of possible
    changes?   3.5 marks

4. Conclusions and summary. Stress what ideas you
have for **2** and **3.**   1 mark

Question 3

You have made the diagnosis of cancer of the lung in a married woman of 66. What arrangements do you make for terminal care?

(*Background:* Much discussion on home care and of terminal care at home and of shared care. You should show that you are aware of problems and that you are experienced in organising this in your own area for your own patients).

Total possible

Answer

1. The disease. It is likely that the life expectancy is about 6–12 months. It is likely that true 'terminal' care will be required only in the last couple of months. Until she is unable to do so she should be encouraged to lead as normal a life as possible.   1 mark

    It is essential that the diagnosis be confirmed by consultant and that management should be a co-operative one.   1 mark

    Main problems are likely to be:
    dyspnoea
    cough
    pain
    weakness   1 mark

2. Family. Someone must be seen and told of diagnosis, of likely course and of plans for management and care.   1 mark

3. Plan of care:
    See regularly – at first consulting room and later at home.   0.5 marks

    Involve the primary care team i.e. nurses, health visitor, social worker, home help, meals on wheels and any other? How, who and when? Manage at home for as long as possible – what indications for hospital/hospice care? How would you arrange admission?   2 marks

*Total
possible*

4. Clinical problems.
  What do you tell patient?
  How do you treat:
    breathlessness?
    pain?
    cough?   1.5 marks

5. Bereavement. Your duty does not cease with death. What arrangements for support and care of relatives?   1 mark

6. Summary and conclusions. Stress roles of GP and his team. Show that you appreciate the problems and that you know how you would mobilise the resources for home care.   1 mark

Answers to Mock MCQ

1.(M)
- **A.** FALSE. Infected milk.
- **B.** FALSE. Recurrent not persistent.
- **C.** TRUE. Correct statement.
- **D.** TRUE. Without serious general ill health.
- **E.** TRUE. Also streptomycin.

2.(T)
- **A.** FALSE. No evidence for this.
- **B.** TRUE. Very important.
- **C.** TRUE. Possibly with drowsiness and depression.
- **D.** TRUE. Guanethidine, bethanidine, debrisoquine and clonidine.
- **E.** TRUE. Can get rebound hypertension.

3.(Ps)
- **A.** FALSE. No evidence for this.
- **B.** FALSE. Blackouts are periods of amnesia.
- **C.** TRUE. From B vitamin deficiency.
- **D.** TRUE. Though commoner in males.
- **E.** FALSE. Must remain total abstainers.

4.(O)
- **A.** TRUE. Standard FPA advice.
- **B.** TRUE. Risk of death from circulatory diseases much increased.
- **C.** FALSE. Risk increases with duration of use.
- **D.** FALSE. Risk not related to duration of use.
- **E.** FALSE. No connection.

5.(M)

A. FALSE. Females more than males.

B. TRUE. 10% of primary myxoedemas have PA.

C. TRUE. Progressive mental dulling then dementia.

D. FALSE. Characteristically shows reduced jerk with delayed return.

E. FALSE. Minimum of lifelong therapy.

6.(CM)

A. TRUE. One reason for psychiatric wards in general hospitals.

B. FALSE. Nearest relative, not any relative, except in emergency (under Section 29).

C. TRUE. Then under Section 26 if further treatment required.

D. FALSE. Can examine the patient within 1 week of each other.

E. TRUE. See **B.**

7.(Ps)

A. TRUE. Unfortunately the GP is often in a position to have the anger and blame directed at him.

B. TRUE. Often self-blame for acts of omission or commission concerning the deceased.

C. TRUE. For about 6 months on average.

D. FALSE. Idealisation.

E. TRUE. Shading over of grief reaction into a frank depressive illness has considerable risk of suicide.

8.(ENT)

A. TRUE. Should be looked for.

B. TRUE. Over all age groups.

C. TRUE. Ambient noise is not being detected by the poor hearing ear.

D. FALSE. Air conduction will still be better than bone conduction which is a positive Rinne.

E. TRUE. Avoids unnecessary amplification.

9.(O)

A. FALSE. 120 ml.

B. TRUE. For any length of cycle.

C. TRUE. Because of increased progesterone.

D. FALSE. No effect.

E. TRUE. Although also high correlation with neuroticism.

10.(M)

A. FALSE. Rapid.

B. TRUE. Lower motor neurone lesion.

C. TRUE. If nerve affected in proximal part of canal.

D. TRUE. Motor effect only.

E. FALSE. May help if given at start.

11.(T)

A. FALSE. Nonsense.

B. TRUE. Inhibits sympathetic activity which occurs with emotion or exercise and prevents cardiac over-activity.

C. FALSE. May cause bronchospasm in the asthmatic.

D. FALSE. May precipitate cardiac failure if there is limited cardiac reserve.

E. TRUE. As B.

12.(Ps)

A. FALSE. Marriage appears to protect men from depression but has a detrimental effect on women.

B. TRUE. Flu, glandular fever etc.

C. TRUE. This is so.

D. TRUE. Hallucinations and mania or catatonia.

E. TRUE. Sedative effect occurs within 1–2 days.

13.(Su)

A. FALSE. 3 to 1 women to men.

B. FALSE. DVT is, but varicose veins *per se* are not.

C. TRUE. Can delineate incompetence.

D. TRUE. Compression sclerotherapy.

E. TRUE. Especially when there has been saphenofemoral incompetence.

14.(M)

   A. FALSE. Aura is caused by this. Subsequent vasodilatation gives headache.

   B. FALSE. No relation to class, intellect or occupation.

   C. TRUE. Aura, unilateral headache and nausea correlate best with diagnosis.

   D. TRUE. After 20–30 years of attacks.

   E. TRUE. Initially a chance finding.

15.(O)

   A. TRUE. Especially in youngsters.

   B. FALSE. Every 24–30 months.

   C. TRUE. Diaphragm pregnancy rate is 3 per 100 woman years (coils 2–5).

   D. TRUE. Coitus interruptus pregnancy rate is 10–17 per 100 woman years (rhythm 14–32).

   E. TRUE. Rarely and one reason for careful selection of cases

16.(Ps)

   A. TRUE. Diurnal variation.

   B. TRUE. Important because may lead to suicide attempts.

   C. FALSE. Not present.

   D. TRUE. Very common.

   E. FALSE. Patient retains insight.

17.(D)

   A. TRUE. This produces the comedo or blackhead.

   B. FALSE. Equally affected.

   C. TRUE. Thought to be because of increased sunshine in the south.

   D. TRUE. If given for weeks or months.

   E. FALSE. Degreasing agents should be used instead of soap and water.

18.(M)

   A. FALSE. 15–35.

   B. TRUE. Dominant with incomplete penetrance.

   C. TRUE. Well known.

   D. TRUE. Especially incompetence.

   E. FALSE. Significant risk of leukaemia.

19.(CM)

  A. FALSE. Morbidity or 'at risk' register for this.

  B. TRUE. Can match for age and sex.

  C. FALSE. Completely inappropriate.

  D. TRUE. Useful for any screening in particular age groups.

  E. TRUE. Obvious.

20.(Ps)

  A. FALSE. Dramatic and sudden.

  B. TRUE. Highly suggestible.

  C. TRUE. They can.

  D. FALSE. Glove and stocking distribution.

  E. FALSE. Not malingering and not consciously aware of motives.

21.(Pa)

  A. TRUE. That is so.

  B. FALSE. From 2 years.

  C. FALSE. Achievement of a new stage depends on the growing maturity of the nervous system so cannot be accelerated by outside sources.

  D. FALSE. Uniform retardation does, but if in single field then first must exclude organic disease, e.g. speech retardation – deafness.

  E. FALSE. Variable.

22.(M)

  A. TRUE. Though once established quite a small food intake can maintain it.

  B. TRUE. Actuarial analysis shows this.

  C. TRUE. Underventilation leads to cor pulmonale.

  D. TRUE. Maturity onset diabetes.

  E. TRUE. Weight watchers etc.

23.(O)

  A. FALSE. Nearly 10%.

  B. TRUE. Fact.

  C. FALSE. Characteristically present with menorrhagia which is increased loss but at normally spaced intervals.

D. TRUE. Observation only.
E. FALSE. How?

24.(Ps)

A. TRUE. Do not adapt to reality.
B. FALSE. Violence is virtually reflex with little or no pre-meditation.
C. FALSE. No guilt or remorse is characteristic.
D. TRUE. Also a few are XYY.
E. TRUE. Complex medicosocial problem.
      Need special units as disrupt everyone else.

25.(Pa)

A. TRUE. ⎫
B. TRUE. ⎪
C. TRUE. ⎬ Straightforward.
D. TRUE. ⎪
E. FALSE. 24 months. ⎭

26.(M)

A. FALSE. Below.
B. TRUE. Especially menorrhagia.
C. TRUE. This is so.
D. FALSE. May be with PA.
E. FALSE. Iron-binding capacity is increased.

27.(T)

A. TRUE. Also crush features of the vertebrae.
B. TRUE. Although euphoria occurs more often.
C. TRUE. Also perforation of an existing ulcer.
D. FALSE. Oestrogen effect.
E. TRUE. Interferes with protein metabolism.

28.(Su)

A. TRUE. Round about puberty especially.
B. TRUE. If any doubt treat as torsion.
C. TRUE. Can get necrosis within 4 hours.
D. TRUE. Correct statement.
E. FALSE. May well make matters worse.

29.(Pa)

   A. FALSE. Equal.
   B. TRUE. Also less fat but more carbohydrate.
   C. FALSE. More.
   D. FALSE. Less.
   E. TRUE. That is so.

30.(M)

   A. FALSE. Exercise should help.
   B. TRUE. Better late than never.
   C. FALSE. No real evidence for this.
   D. FALSE. Of no possible benefit to the patient.
   E. FALSE. Nonsense.

31.(Op)

   A. TRUE. Infants and young children are very rarely myopic.
   B. FALSE. Very important confirmatory test.
   C. TRUE. Early referral is important.
   D. TRUE. Also convex spectacles to correct any hypermetropia.
   E. FALSE. Sensory exercises to help develop stereoscopic vision.

32.(Ps)

   A. FALSE. Apathetic but clearly orientated.
   B. FALSE. Normal.
   C. TRUE. From failure of affect.
   D. TRUE. Easy.
   E. TRUE. Ideas of reference.

33.(O)

   A. FALSE. 49–50 now.
   B. FALSE. Rises if anything.
   C. TRUE. Hot flushes.
   D. TRUE. Risk of endometrial carcinoma.
   E. TRUE. Strong circumstantial evidence of this.

34.(M)

A. TRUE. DU is commoner in men.

B. TRUE. GU is commoner in 4 + 5.

C. FALSE. Decreased.

D. TRUE. 85% are on lesser curvature.

E. TRUE. Though strangely not before breakfast.

35.(Pa)

A. FALSE. As yet no evidence for this.

B. TRUE. Sudden infant death is associated with bottle feeding.

C. TRUE. Inhibits ovulation.

D. TRUE. This is so.

E. FALSE. Human milk has adequate Vitamin C.

36.(Ps)

A. FALSE. Amenorrhoea.

B. FALSE. Typically hyperactive.

C. TRUE. Imagine themselves to be fatter than they actually are.

D. TRUE. Especially at start of illness.

E. TRUE. Usually from laxative abuse.

37.(Op)

A. TRUE. These are clumps of pus cells adhering to the back of the cornea.

B. FALSE. Either not affected or constricted because of associated iritis.

C. TRUE, Tarsal conjuctiva is affected as well.

D. TRUE. Are of enormous value.

E. FALSE. Miotics.

38.(M)

A. FALSE. 3 years fit-free.

B. TRUE. Remember this.

C. TRUE. Need exercise ECG.

D. FALSE. More than 10^5 for diagnosis.

E. FALSE. Not appropriate in this context.

39.(Ps)
- **A.** FALSE. Constipation.
- **B.** TRUE. Incriminated as possible factor in deaths of patients with cardiac disease.
- **C.** TRUE. May be a drug reaction or because of relief of depression.
- **D.** FALSE. Sedative properties allay this.
- **E.** TRUE. Atropine like effect.

40.(ENT)
- **A.** FALSE. The opposite is the case.
- **B.** TRUE. This is a correct statement.
- **C.** FALSE. May be so severe that the patient will lie still on the ground because he is scared to move but no loss of consciousness.
- **D.** TRUE. An audiometric test.
- **E.** TRUE. Also promethazine or beta histine (Serc).

41.(CM)
- **A.** TRUE. Headache, anxiety, depression, etc. are symptoms rather than precise labels.
- **B.** TRUE. Easily doubted at the end of a long surgery!
- **C.** FALSE. Second to respiratory disorders.
- **D.** TRUE. Sad to say.
- **E.** TRUE. 'Catarrhal child'.

42.(M)
- **A.** FALSE. Fine tremor. Coarse tremor suggests anxiety.
- **B.** TRUE. Common.
- **C.** FALSE. Atrial fibrillation in 5–10%.
- **D.** TRUE. May need steroids or orbital decompression.
- **E.** FALSE. Myxoedema will develop and need treatment.

43.(T)
- **A.** FALSE. No effect in acute situation.
- **B.** TRUE. Vital to know this.
- **C.** FALSE. Must be switched to oral or parenteral corticosteroids.
- **D.** FALSE. Why should it be?
- **E.** TRUE. Especially with excessive use of the aerosol preparation.

44.(O)

A. TRUE. pH5–6.5.
B. TRUE. More acid and carbohydrate.
C. TRUE. Well known.
D. TRUE. Opportunistic infection.
E. TRUE. Though usually white and cheesy.

45.(Su)

A. TRUE. No significant alteration in last 20 years.
B. TRUE. Also is age 35-plus at first pregnancy.
C. TRUE. From well-differentiated to anaplastic.
D. FALSE. Generally self-diagnosed painless lump.
E. TRUE. Least mutilatory operation is preferable.

46.(M)

A. TRUE. They are.
B. FALSE. By stooping or lying flat.
C. TRUE. Can give chronic bleeding.
D. FALSE. Head raised helps.
E. TRUE. It does.

47.(Ps)

A. TRUE. Unable to form normal emotional relationships.
B. TRUE. That is so.
C. TRUE. One-third are mute.
D. FALSE. The reverse.
E. FALSE. No connection.

48.(Pa)

A. TRUE. Symptoms only if reach anus.
B. FALSE. Hookworm can.
C. FALSE. Think of life cycle.
D. FALSE. All affected.
E. TRUE. 90% cure rate.

49.(O)

A. TRUE. In 50–60%.
B. FALSE. Pain then bleeding.
C. TRUE. Caused by blood tracking to the diaphragm.

D. TRUE. Negative physical signs should not be allowed to overrule symptoms.

E. FALSE. Does not tell you if intra- or extra-uterine pregnancy, and in 50% of cases is negative because the chorionic tissue is dead.

50.(M)
A. FALSE. No connection.
B. TRUE. It is.
C. FALSE. Not if uncomplicated.
D. TRUE. Frequently.
E. FALSE. Unless complicated by empyema or lung abscess.

51.(Ps)
A. TRUE. As one would expect.
B. FALSE. Greatly affected.
C. TRUE. Also lessened in Ulster at present.
D. TRUE. 40% will have seen their GP within the previous 2 weeks.
E. TRUE. Increasing incidence but decreasing mortality.

52.(CM)
A. TRUE. If vital then can be given at same time as far apart on the body as possible.
B. TRUE. Reaction most likely from the whooping cough component.
C. FALSE. For 2 months.
D. FALSE. Tuberculin negative.
E. FALSE. 6 days.

53.(T)
A. TRUE. That is why potassium supplements are used.
B. TRUE. This is how diuretics work.
C. FALSE. The reverse is the case.
D. TRUE. Usually resolves when the diuretic is stopped.
E. FALSE. 12 hours.

54.(M)
A. TRUE. Random mutation may account for the rest.
B. TRUE. Get a Y from their father, not an X.

C. FALSE. Half would.

D. FALSE. Factor 9 deficiency is Christmas disease.

E. TRUE. Correct.

55.(Ps)

A. FALSE. Reality has the same meaning as for the rest of the community.

B. TRUE. Easy.

C. FALSE. Quite the reverse.

D. FALSE. Mental conflict exists which therapy tries to make obvious to the patient.

E. TRUE. Free floating or related to specific situations.

56.(O)

A. TRUE. CDH, talipes, hydrocephaly.

B. TRUE. Cleft lip.

C. TRUE. Goitre and cretinism.

D. FALSE. No evidence.

E. TRUE. Masculinisation of female fetus.

57.(Pa)

A. TRUE. Be suspicious.

B. TRUE. Twisting injury.

C. FALSE. Any social class.

D. FALSE. If only it were true.

E. TRUE. Often essential to confirm diagnosis.

58.(M)

A. TRUE. About 3% of the population in total.

B. FALSE. Increases it.

C. FALSE. 16 units.

D. TRUE. Soluble and Lente cannot be mixed.

E. FALSE. AND CRIMINAL!

59.(Op)

A. TRUE. Generally 50+ at onset.

B. FALSE. Hypermetropes, because they have shallower anterior chamber.

C. TRUE. Cataract/senile degeneration of the macula and glaucoma are the three main causes of blindness.

D. TRUE. Correct statement.

E. TRUE. Miotics are the first line of treatment.

60.(T)

A. TRUE. 80% is finally excreted in the urine.

B. FALSE. The opposite is the case.

C. TRUE. Long half-life.

D. TRUE. Usually because of impaired renal function.

E. FALSE. This is an indication for using digoxin.

62.(M)

A. TRUE. Except Japan.

B. FALSE. Commoner in 1 + 2 like polio.

C. TRUE. This can remain the only symptom.

D. TRUE. This is so.

E. TRUE. Also depression commonly in the other two-thirds.

61.(D)

A. FALSE. Mainly young people.

B. TRUE. Herald patch.

C. TRUE. Usually ceases at upper thighs and upper arms.

D. FALSE. Probably viral.

E. FALSE. 6 weeks to 3 months.

63.(Ps)

A. FALSE. Recent memory lost first.

B. TRUE. Time first then place and person.

C. TRUE. Also lose control of emotions.

D. FALSE. Not at all.

E. FALSE. Unfortunately not.

64.(O)

A. TRUE. Distends uterus.

B. TRUE. 50% are premature.

C. TRUE. Accounts for 12% premature labours.

D. FALSE. No connection.

E. TRUE. Either stillbirth or intervention.

65.(Pa)

A. FALSE. Males more than females.

B. FALSE. Earlier than this.

C. FALSE. Avid for food.

D. TRUE. May see reverse peristalsis, projectile vomiting or feel pyloric tumour.

E. TRUE. Highly effective operation.

66.(M)

A. TRUE. By oedema or fatty material.

B. TRUE. Also myxoedema or obesity.

C. FALSE. This is ulnar distribution.

D. TRUE. Especially scrubbing or washing clothes.

E. TRUE. Can be helped by a splint at night.

67.(Ps)

A. TRUE. Also other heavy metals.

B. FALSE. No connection.

C. FALSE. No connection.

D. TRUE. Primary or secondary.

E. TRUE. Well known.

68.(Su)

A. TRUE. This is so.

B. FALSE. Can occur but Fe deficiency far commoner.

C. TRUE. Both patient and doctor can be lulled and delay presentation or investigation.

D. FALSE. High roughage.

E. FALSE. Bilirubin in urine not urobilinogen.

69.(Pa)

A. FALSE. Irrelevant.

B. TRUE. Correct.

C. FALSE. Irrelevant.

D. TRUE. Correct.

E. TRUE. Correct.

70.(M)

A. FALSE. Think of physiology of CVS.

B. TRUE. Stage 2 of hypertensive retinopathy.

C. FALSE. Only indicated if some suggestion of renal abnormality.

D. FALSE. Unrealistic. Aim to get diastolic below 100.
E. TRUE. Recognised side-effect.

71.(D)
A. TRUE. Most important aetiological factor is heredity.
B. TRUE. Gives acute guttate psoriasis.
C. FALSE. Pitting etc in 25% of cases.
D. TRUE. Mild cases may clear after 3 weeks but severe cases require up to 6 weeks.
E. TRUE. Will either reappear during treatment or relapse with greater severity when stopped.

72.(T)
A. TRUE. Similarity with aspirin overdoses.
B. FALSE. No gastric side-effects.
C. TRUE. In hospital.
D. FALSE. Dangerous course of action in view of **E.**
E. TRUE. Important to know this.

73.(ENT)
A. FALSE. Probably less than 50%.
B. TRUE. Two out of three will have more than one attack.
C. FALSE. Contraindicated in children and pregnancy.
D. FALSE. All patients should be seen in 2–3 weeks to check drum and hearing.
E. FALSE. Can give glue ear or damage to ossicles.

74.(M)
A. FALSE. No evidence for this.
B. TRUE. If below 100 litres per minute then patient is in serious trouble.
C. FALSE. Why should it?
D. FALSE. Prolonged expiration.
E. TRUE. Well known. Also mesothelioma.

75.(Ps)
A. FALSE. They are words of the patient's own making.
B. TRUE. 'Cocaine bug.'
C. TRUE. Unlike stereotypy which is monotonous repetition of an action.

D. FALSE. That is an hallucination. Illusions are based on misinterpretation of external stimuli.

E. TRUE. Type of automatic behaviour.

76.(O)

A. TRUE. At 30 weeks one in four fetuses are breech.

B. FALSE. Normal version occurs at 34 weeks, while engagement of the head does not occur until some time after.

C. FALSE. Why should it?

D. TRUE. Prevents version.

E. TRUE. As D.

77.(Pa)

A. FALSE. Increases and only subsides as rash fades.

B. FALSE. This is smallpox.

C. TRUE. Correct.

D. FALSE. First day.

E. FALSE. Glandular fever.

78.(T)

A. TRUE. Applies to all age groups.

B. FALSE. Smaller doses, with build-up if no side-effects, is a safer method.

C. TRUE. Hypotension and hypothermia may develop.

D. FALSE. Both symptoms and side-effects are increased in the elderly, so better to keep prescribing at a minimum.

E. TRUE. As **D.**

79.(CM)

A. TRUE. Wives and children take husbands' class.

B. FALSE. Occupation, not income, is criterion.

C. FALSE. 5.

D. TRUE. Useful research tool.

E. FALSE. All doctors class 1.

80.(Pa)

A. FALSE. Certainly not.

B. TRUE. In about 1 in 20.

C. FALSE. No sedative effect.
D. FALSE. Rare.
E. TRUE. Current stress or unhappiness though should do MSSU to exclude infection.

81.(Ps)
A. TRUE. Women at late 30s.
B. TRUE. Practised by nearly all persons of both sexes at some time in their lives.
C. TRUE. It has.
D. FALSE. Only male homosexuality is punishable.
E. FALSE. Dramatic response to treatment 98% cure in 2 weeks by Masters and Johnson.

82.(M)
A. FALSE. All ages.
B. TRUE. 30 times.
C. TRUE. Especially chronic myeloid.
D. TRUE. Due to thrombosis of the corpora cavernosa.
E. TRUE. One-third are aleukaemic with lowered WBC, RBC and platelets.

83.(O)
A. TRUE. If not, think of ectopic.
B. TRUE. XO, triploidy and trisomy especially.
C. FALSE. Increased fetal mortality.
D. FALSE. Habitual abortion. Cervical incompetence occurs later than this.
E. TRUE. Also after pregnancy or hydatidiform mole.

84.(T)
A. FALSE. It has none at all.
B. TRUE. Gradual withdrawal better.
C. FALSE. It has frequent and serious toxic effects.
D. FALSE. 3 months or more before get effect.
E. TRUE. Applies to many anti-inflammatory drugs.

85.(D)
A. FALSE. Rarely may give erythema multiforme.
B. TRUE. Important cause.

C. FALSE. Common cause of erythema multiforme.

D. TRUE. Especially in children, and must not assume history of previous sore throat rules out TB.

E. TRUE. Commonest cause.

86.(Ps)

A. FALSE. Often at adolescence with maximum incidence in 20s.

B. FALSE. Genetic factors are most important.

C. TRUE. Nearly two-thirds.

D. FALSE. This is phobic anxiety.

E. TRUE. Although not always.

87.(Su)

A. FALSE. Certainly not.

B. TRUE. Very important.

C. TRUE. Well recognised.

D. FALSE. No evidence of this.

E. TRUE. 20% develop malignant change.

88.(O)

A. FALSE. PET occurs in the second half of pregnancy. Suspect a mole.

B. FALSE. Risks greater than any possible benefit.

C. TRUE. Correct statement.

D. TRUE. Especially in prims.

E. FALSE. Engages with labour.

89.(T)

A. FALSE. Occurs in about 7% of patients.

B. TRUE. Reason why its use is generally restricted.

C TRUE. Both vestibular and auditory divisions can be affected.

D. TRUE. Use with caution in the elderly.

E. TRUE. Hepatocellular or cholestatic.

90.(Ps)
    A. FALSE. This is its main side-effect.
    B. TRUE. It can.
    C. TRUE. In 1–2%.
    D. TRUE. Can be very effective.
    E. TRUE. It is.